T5-CRZ-576

DATE DUE

| | | | |
|---|---|---|---|
| | | | |
| | | | |
| | | | |
| | | | |
| | | | |
| | | | |
| | | | |
| | | | |
| | | | |
| | | | |
| | | | |
| | | | |
| | | | |

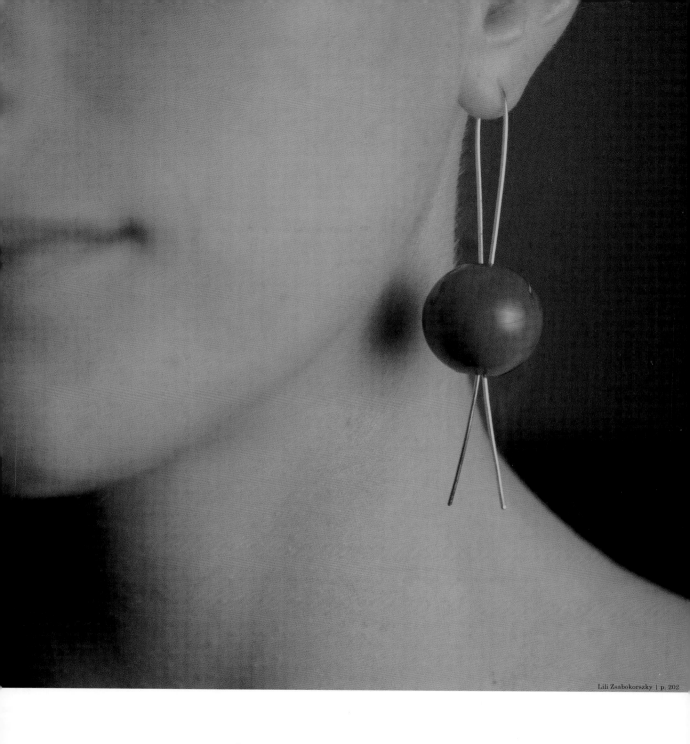

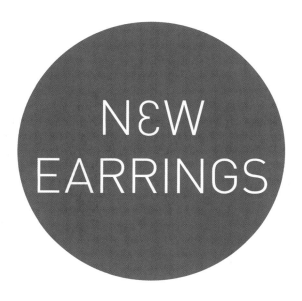

# NEW EARRINGS

## 500+ DESIGNS FROM AROUND THE WORLD

### Nicolas Estrada

with 530 color illustrations

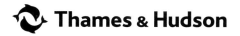

Thames & Hudson

On the cover:
*Front:* 'Calota' by Anne Bader.
*Back, clockwise from top left:* 'Yellow Lemons' by Mareen Alburg
Duncker; 'Basket Weir' by Jan Smith; 'Africanas' by Roc Majoral
and Abril Ribera; 'Untitled' by Ferran Iglesias.

Translated from the Spanish *Pendientes: 500 creaciones artísticas
de todo el mundo* by Satèl·lit bcn – Hugo Steckelmacher.

First published in the United Kingdom in 2013 by
Thames & Hudson Ltd, 181A High Holborn, London WC1V 7QX

www.thamesandhudson.com

First published in 2013 in paperback in the United States of
America by Thames & Hudson Inc., 500 Fifth Avenue, New York,
New York 10110

thamesandhudsonusa.com

Original edition © 2013 Promopress, Barcelona
This edition © 2013 Thames & Hudson Ltd, London

Author: Nicolas Estrada
Introductory texts: Noel Guyomarc'h and Carolina Hornauer

British Library Cataloguing-in-Publication Data
A catalogue record for this book is available from the British
Library

Library of Congress Catalog Card Number 2012946302

ISBN: 978-0-500-29082-8

Printed and bound in China

# CONTENTS

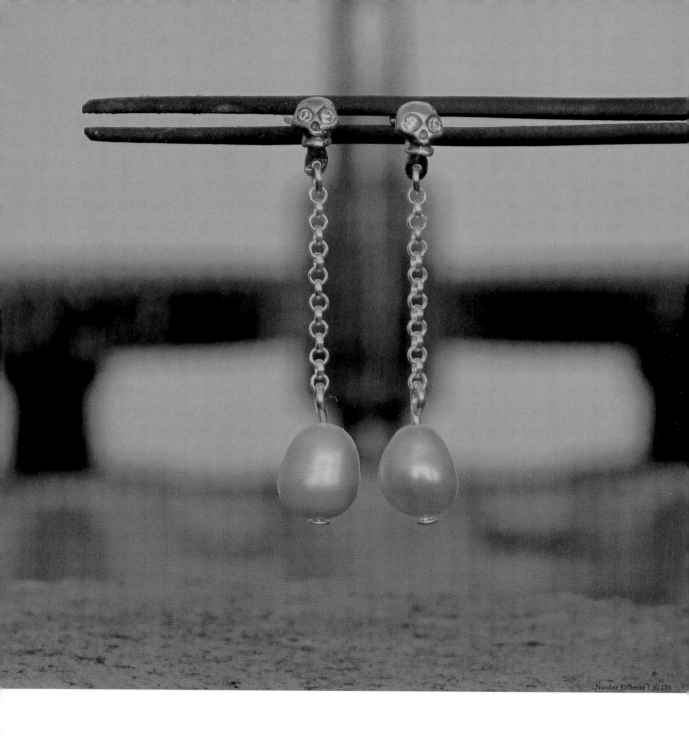

# NICOLAS ESTRADA

**About the Author**

Every piece of jewelry
draws the viewer into a
story and a world of its own.

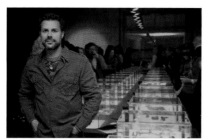

Photo: Līga Ērkšķe

In Nicolas Estrada we find an artist who possesses a strong, individual voice and a bold artistic vision that combines delicate irony and acute insight. With the passion of a craftsman forging new interpretations, his works are driven by an inexorable current, a flow that pushes him to use a broad but harmonious palette of techniques with subtle nuances.

Born in Medellín, Colombia, Nicolas came to Barcelona as a businessman, but his career path changed dramatically when he discovered his true calling: to create unique jewelry with a story to tell. He launched himself into the study of a wide variety of jewelry techniques at the Massana School in Barcelona. A promising student, he soon won awards from Enjoia't, Swarovski and the Marzee Gallery, paving the way for things to come. He has since built on this foundation with courses on various techniques, all around the world.

Nicolas held his first solo show, 'Dos Mundos', at the Magari Gallery in Barcelona in 2004. His first venture in the United States took place in the same year at San Francisco's Velvet da Vinci Gallery. After numerous exhibitions in various countries in Europe, the US and South America,

Nicolas had a major breakthrough when he exhibited at Barcelona's Maritime Museum in 2007, heralding his transition from jewelry-maker to bona fide artist. He was most recently showcased at 'Think Again: New Latin American Jewelry' at New York's Museum of Art and Design (MAD), marking him out as one of the outstanding Latin American jewelers of our time.

The author of *New Rings: 500+ Designs from Around the World* (2011), Nicolas has consolidated his reputation as an innovative, conceptually aware designer with contributions to many international magazines and books.

At his atelier, Amarillo Joyas, Nicolas fashions jewelry that shares an intimate bond with its wearer. Depicting images such as a melancholy soldier, hearts enslaved by secret desires or virgins brimming with bitterness, each piece draws the viewer into a story and a world of its own. A thirst for variety and for forging connections with viewers and readers defines both his oeuvre and his relationship with this book, for which he has selected works by a range of the most significant jewelry artists from all over the world, whose pieces speak and inspire.

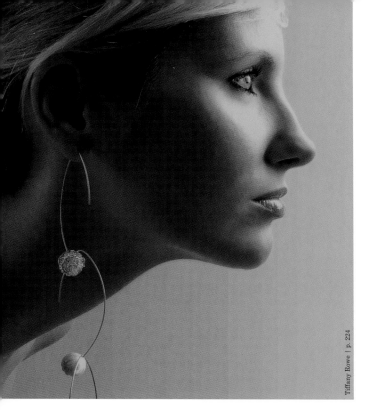

Tiffany Rowe | p. 224

### Noel Guyomarc'h

## Adorning the face, earrings immediately catch the eye when worn.

Bridging the gap between compliment and complement, they convey harmony, at once embellishing and surprising. When you set about making a pair of earrings, many diverse factors must be considered: weight, dimensions, symmetry or lack thereof, balance, repetition, the fluidity of the lines and, of course, design. However, earrings are notable only for their absence in most volumes on contemporary jewelry, with this creative form seemingly relegated to the background behind brooches, necklaces and rings as a field for invention and creation suitable for the craft of art jewelers. Despite remaining some of the most popular jewelry items among wearers, earrings are all too often shunned by artists.

This book draws together a variety of creative approaches and methods. Employing an array of materials, the designs on show range from traditional forms – many with a tribal inspiration – to more complex styles, based on cutting-edge technology. The practical constraints involved in making earrings have become challenges to which the jewelers featured here have responded with ingenuity, flamboyance, elegance, sensitivity and, in many cases, a great deal of freedom.

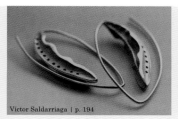

Victor Saldarriaga | p. 194

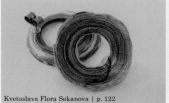

Kvetoslava Flora Sekanova | p. 122

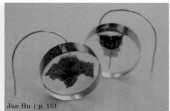

Jun Hu | p. 151

All the pieces featured are notable for their boldness, whether in terms of dimension, colour or composition, their exuberance or the materials selected.

Frequently inspired by conventional earring styles, such as girandoles and studs, some of the creators achieve surprisingly creative results by replacing traditional materials with unexpected ones such as porcelain and plastic. Sometimes, where the material lends itself to this treatment, the artists choose simply to distil and foreground the profile of the piece. Others, meanwhile, continue to make use of classical materials such as gold, silver and gemstones, putting an original, subtle and sophisticated spin on their designs through their decoration, shape, format and the simplicity of their execution. In some cases, the designs are imbued with a theme and a message. Unconventional and occasionally provocative motifs, such as trophies, amulets, charms and items from everyday life, can function as symbols of identity or illustrate contemporary concerns.

Whatever the materials chosen, it is the design that shines through.

Stones are often chosen for their natural colours. Whether cut to shape or left in their rough form, they offer sparkle and lustre, drawing the eye of customers. Many of the earrings showcased here stand out for their ingenuity and refinement. While the quest for aesthetic fulfilment is a fixture throughout the designs in this book, there is also room for exploration and play. Innovation takes centre stage. The use of enamel, plastic, laminates and felt affords a number of possibilities for fashioning new colour palettes, textures and unusual forms. A mixture of simple and complex lines establishes an interplay between positive and negative space, light and shadow, while retaining the sense of harmony and surprise. Asymmetry gives rise to original flourishes, as the two earrings dovetail, respond to and probe one another, coming to a sort of balance in spite (or by virtue) of their differences. The miscellaneous approaches displayed in this book highlight the inexhaustible creative potential offered by earrings.

# PREFACE

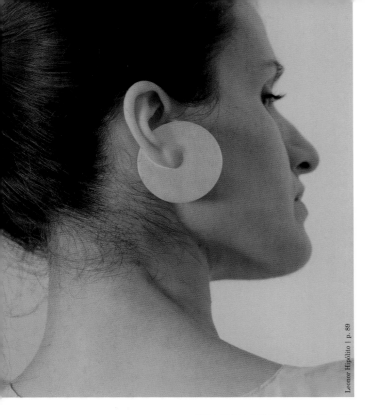

Leonor Hipólito | p. 89

# INDELIBLE MARKS

**Carolina Hornauer**

The ear is the organ responsible for detecting sound and maintaining our balance.

Since around 3000 BC, this delicate shell of cartilage has also been used to display earrings of all kinds. These little objects can symbolize everything from ethnic group to class, gender, personal idiosyncrasies, age and wealth. This member of the jewelry family has proven itself the most independent with regards to its wearer, as it hangs off the body and needs only a small element to fix it in place. It may even dangle away from its owner, hovering between the face and neck, a position that allows it – unlike other jewelry – to reveal both its front and rear sides. And, as if that weren't enough, it also leaves indelible marks on our ears.

Before attaining enlightenment and gaining recognition as Shakyamuni Buddha, the young Siddhartha Gautama was an affluent Nepalese prince. According to the customs of his time and culture, men showed off their wealth by adorning their earlobes with an abundance of ornaments in precious metal and gemstones. As the story goes, the prince followed this tradition, living in a palace and upholding his position of power and noble rank from his early childhood to the age of twenty-nine. But then, curious about what lay outside his royal abode, the prince decided to leave the palace and take up life as an ascetic and, later, a monk. Though he divested himself of all of his worldly riches, his earlobes remained elongated, stretched by the weight of the heavy earrings he once wore.

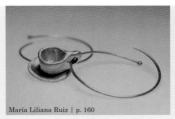

María Liliana Ruiz | p. 160

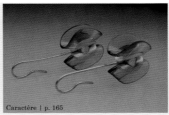

Caractère | p. 165

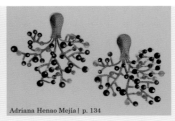

Adriana Henao Mejía | p. 134

For Buddhists, this physical feature embodies the wisdom and the renunciation of the material world that the followers of Gautama Buddha strive towards. These large ears allowed the Buddha to take in the sounds of a world of tears and suffering, to which he responded with boundless compassion.

Besides ranking among the oldest ornaments in human history, earrings have been regarded as capable of drawing together spirituality, the intellect and beauty.

They also ally creativity and the world of sound. Most earrings are fastened to the body through piercings in the ear. As such, they are the only piece of jewelry that, by its nature, indelibly modifies the body in order to embellish it. Just as there are large earrings that can deform or stretch the ear, so the size and design of other pieces identify the wearer with a minimalist aesthetic, verging on the imperceptible: earrings that are delicate and almost invisible, finely crafted to the point of fragility.

If the myth of Buddha removing his earrings paved the way for a whole philosophy and system of symbols, for the Mapuche (an indigenous people from the south of Chile and southwestern Argentina), the ritual of putting on earrings for the first time plays the role of sealing their bond with their culture and differentiating between the genders.

At the event known as the *Katan Pilun'N*, or 'ear-piercing festival', women of the Mapuche community reinforce their kinship with the group and with Mother Earth. The ceremony begins when the Machi (a practitioner of traditional medicine and ritual) calls on the god Ngenechén to bestow prosperity, health and wisdom upon the young girl in whose honour the rite is being held. Using a silver pin, the Machi pierces the girl's ears and sews in a thread of wool which will be removed when the wound heals. This is followed by the attachment of the first earrings, or *chaway*, which represent a magical system that identifies its wearer's gender, protects her and connects her to the land of her forefathers.

As I explored these pieces, I became fully aware of the poetic potential of earrings to channel the voices of our intellect and emotions. It is therefore up to the jewelers themselves to continue making earrings that reveal a language infused with symbolism, sound and vitality. Indeed, contemporary jewelry is a privileged arena for the development of a whole host of new forms of expression, centred around these objects which, despite their humble beginnings as nothing more than small pieces of metal placed through the earlobe, can nonetheless give rise to all manner of genres and styles.

# INTRODUCTION

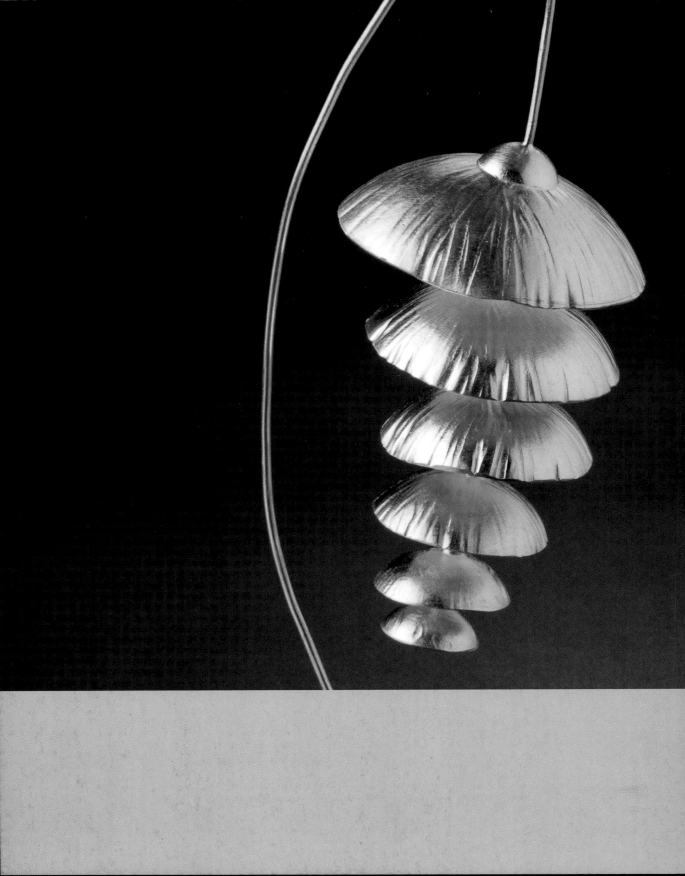

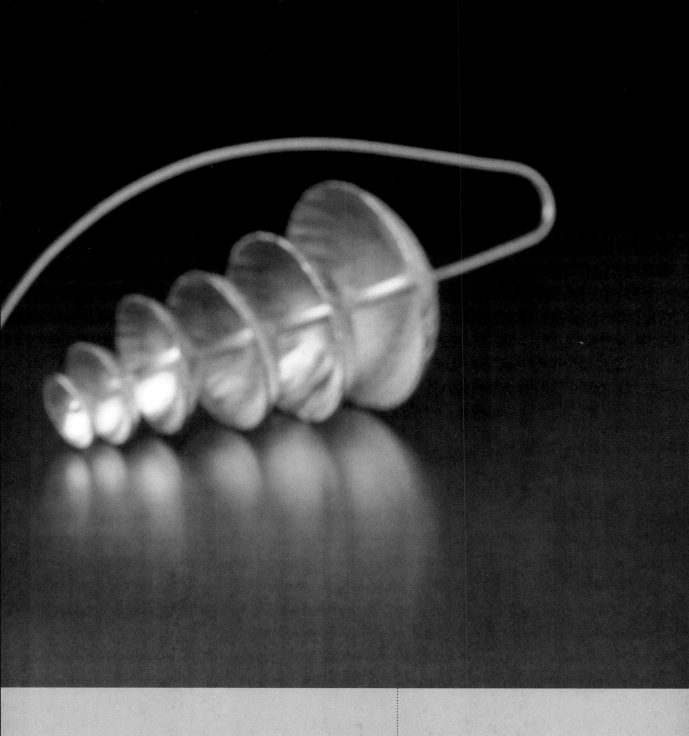

ELEGANT

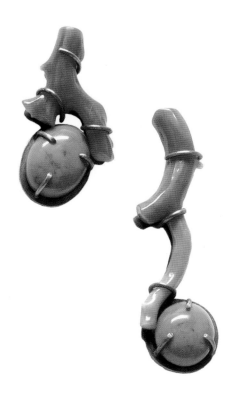

**HUI-MEI PAN**
Co+Tu

Media: 925 silver, natural
undyed coral, turquoise

Photo: Hui-Mei Pan

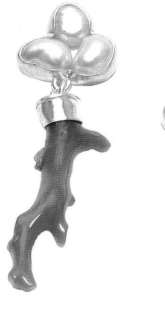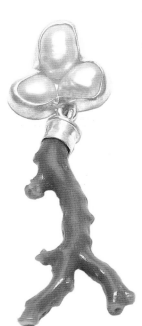

**HUI-MEI PAN**
Pe+Co

Media: 925 silver, natural
undyed coral, pearls

Photo: Hui-Mei Pan

**RIKE BARTELS**
Double Dog Portrait II

..........................................................

Media: 22ct gold, coral

..........................................................

Photo: Jens Mauritz

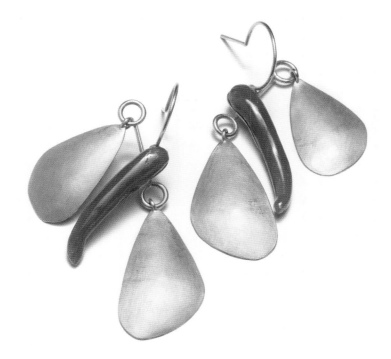

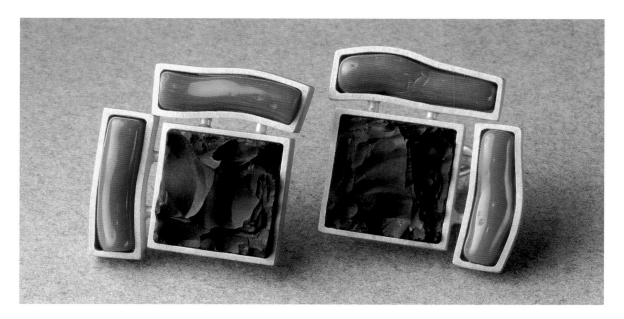

**PILAR GARRIGOSA**
Untitled

..........................................................

Media: 18ct gold, coral, onyx

..........................................................

Photo: Nos y Soto

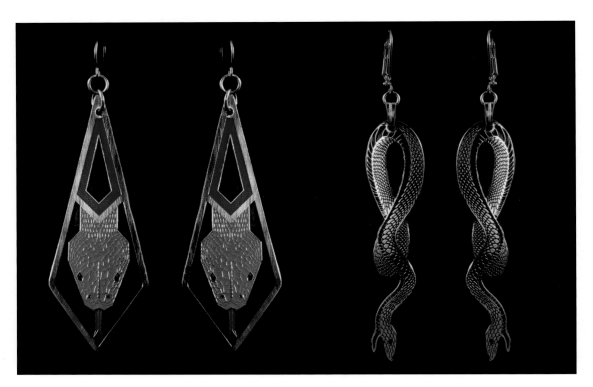

**FEDERICO CASTRILLÓN**
Deco Snakes

Media: photo-engraved stainless steel
leaf, enamel

Photo: Federico Castrillón

**FEDERICO CASTRILLÓN**
Asps

Media: gold-plated photo-engraved
bronze leaf, enamel

Photo: Federico Castrillón

**FEDERICO CASTRILLÓN**
Lynxes

Media: gold-plated photo-engraved
bronze leaf, enamel, crystals

Photo: Federico Castrillón

**FEDERICO CASTRILLÓN**
Swans

Media: photo-engraved stainless steel
leaf, enamel, crystals

Photo: Federico Castrillón

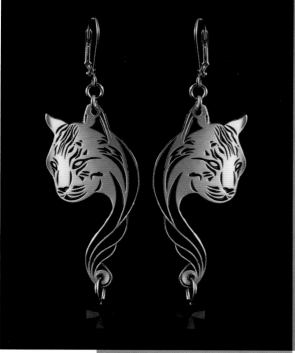

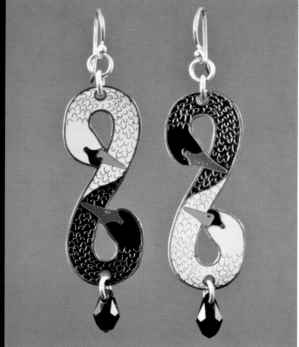

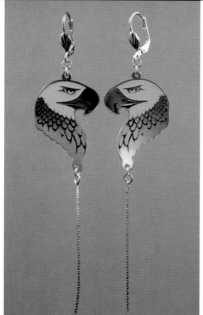

**FEDERICO CASTRILLÓN**
Imperial Eagles

Media: gold-plated photo-engraved
bronze leaf, enamel

Photo: Federico Castrillón

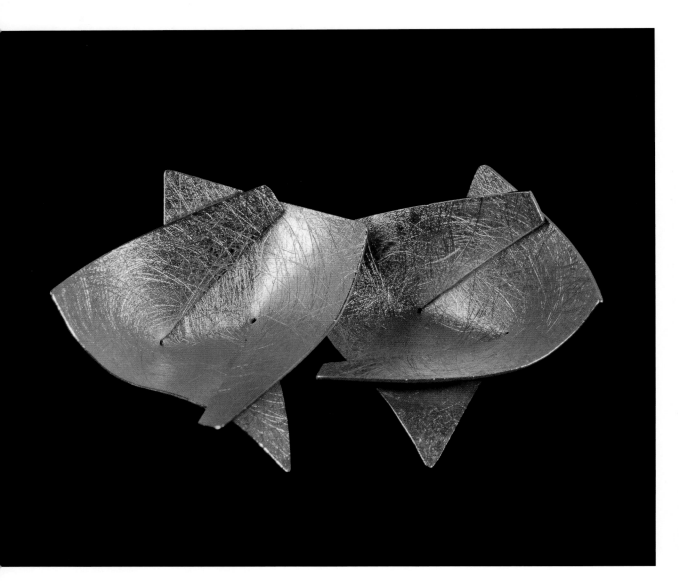

**MIGUEL GASSÓ**
Folds – Conguiteras

Medium: 18ct gold

Photo: Rieragassó

**SALVADOR MALLOL**
Diabolo

Media: gold, steel

Photo: Lafotografica

**SALVADOR MALLOL**
Symmetry

Media: silver, nylon

Photo: Lafotografica

**SALVADOR MALLOL**
Purse

Media: gold, steel

Photo: Lafotografica

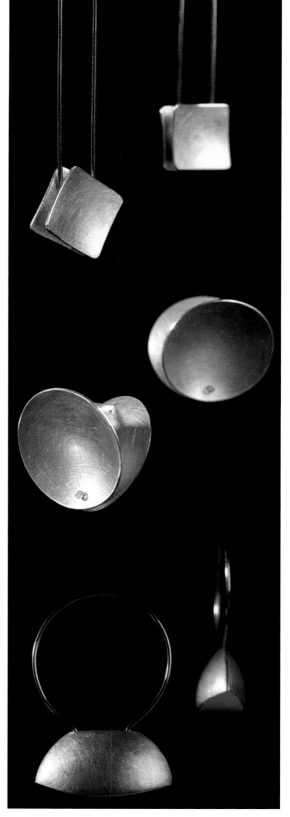

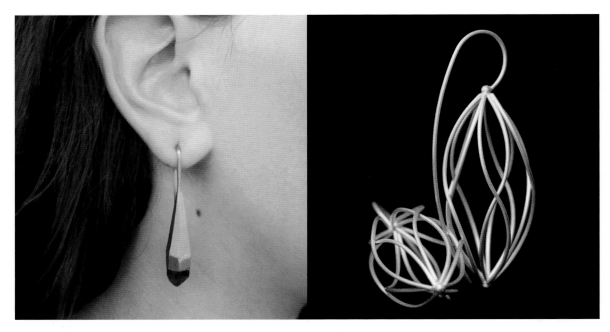

**AINA MINISTRAL**
Chrysalis

Media: 18ct gold, citrine quartz

Photo: Agnés Mora

**FERRAN IGLESIAS**
Untitled

Medium: 18ct gold

Photo: Ferran Iglesias

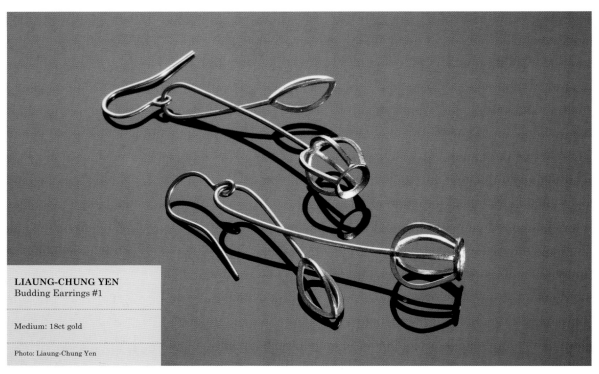

**LIAUNG-CHUNG YEN**
Budding Earrings #1

Medium: 18ct gold

Photo: Liaung-Chung Yen

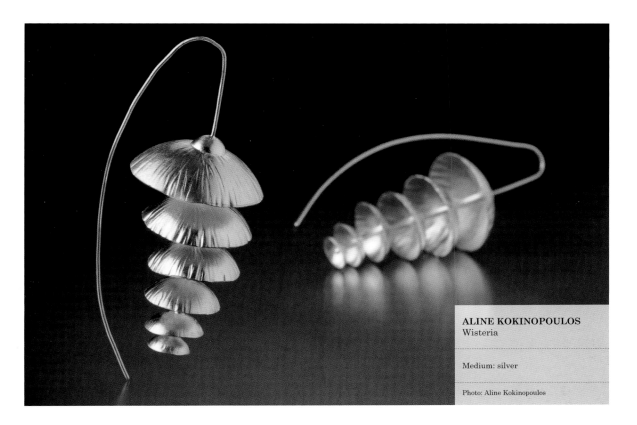

**ALINE KOKINOPOULOS**
Wisteria

Medium: silver

Photo: Aline Kokinopoulos

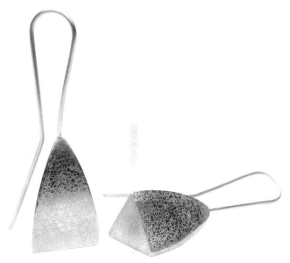

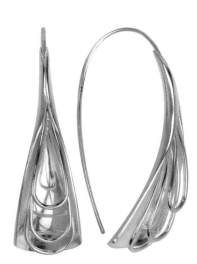

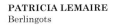

**PATRICIA LEMAIRE**
Berlingots

Medium: 925 guilloché silver

Photo: Ecliptique – Laurent Thion

**MARINA BABIĆ**
Flourishing Earrings

Media: 925 silver, 18ct gold

Photo: Digital by Design – Paul Ambtman

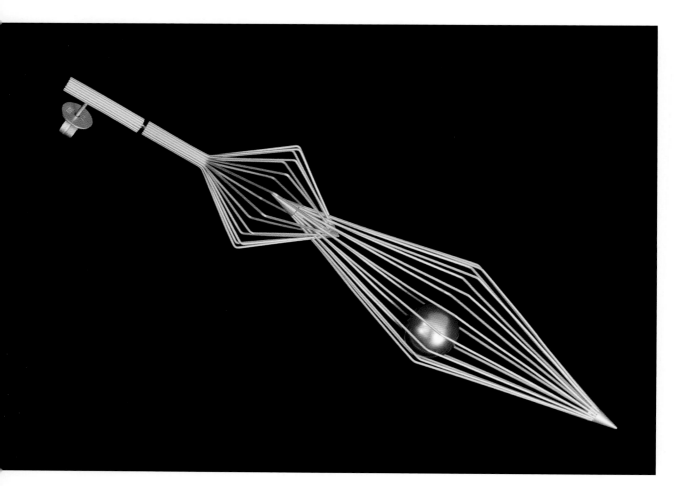

**FERRAN IGLESIAS**
Untitled

Media: 18ct gold, Tahitian pearl

Photo: Ferran Iglesias

**FERRAN IGLESIAS**
Untitled

Medium: 18ct gold

Photo: Ferran Iglesias

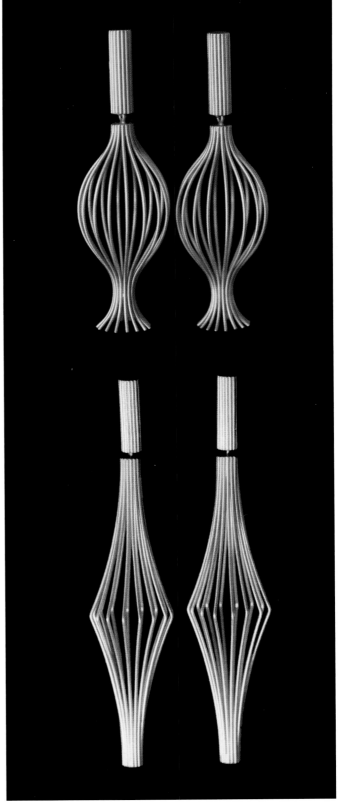

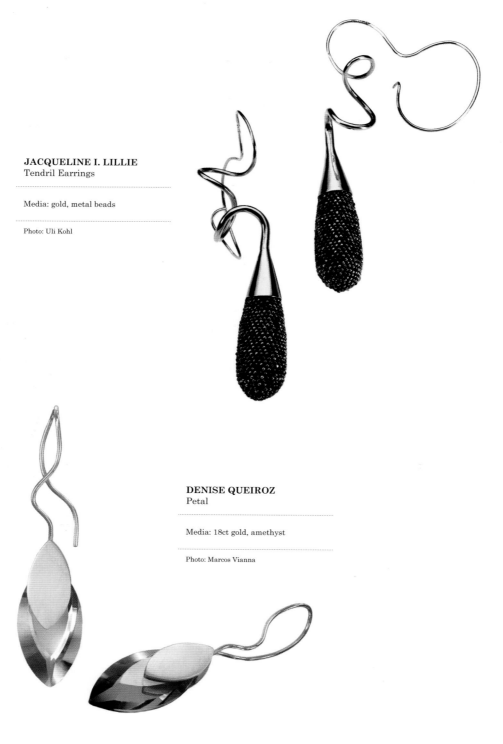

**JACQUELINE I. LILLIE**
Tendril Earrings

Media: gold, metal beads

Photo: Uli Kohl

**DENISE QUEIROZ**
Petal

Media: 18ct gold, amethyst

Photo: Marcos Vianna

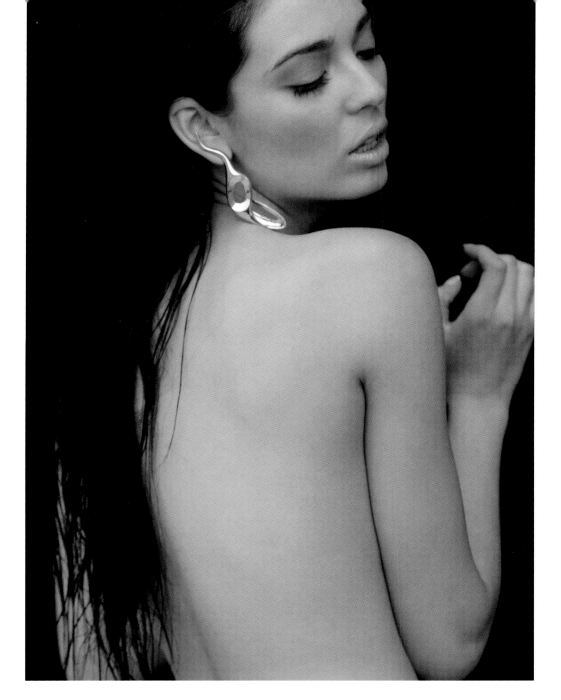

**XANATH LAMMOGLIA
BUSTAMANTE**
Sperma Earrings

Media: 925 silver, rhodium
electroplated

Photo: Álvaro Nates

**LLUÍS DURAN**
Apse

Media: silver, coral

Photo: Lluís Duran

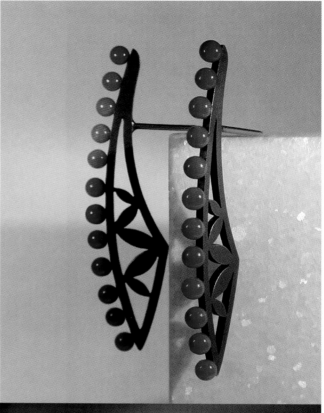

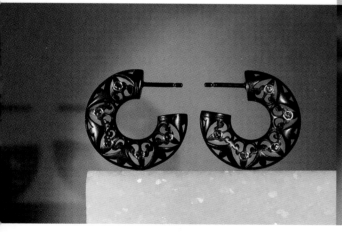

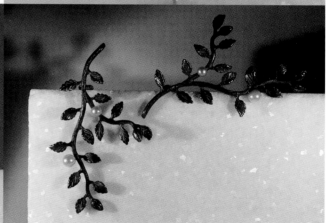

**LLUÍS DURAN**
Openwork

Media: silver, yellow gold, rubies

Photo: Lluís Duran

**LLUÍS DURAN**
Floral

Media: silver, pearls

Photo: Lluís Duran

**MARTHA VARGAS**
Corsage

Media: silver, gold, inlaid wood

Photo: Martha Vargas

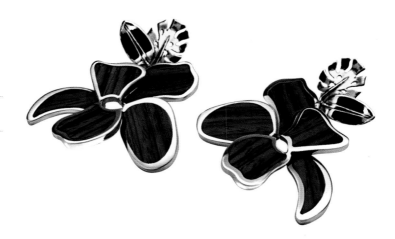

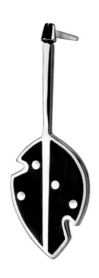
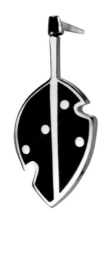

**MARTHA VARGAS**
Silver Drops

Medium: silver with wood inlay

Photo: Martha Vargas

**MARTHA VARGAS**
Tiger's Claw

Media: silver with wood inlay

Photo: Martha Vargas

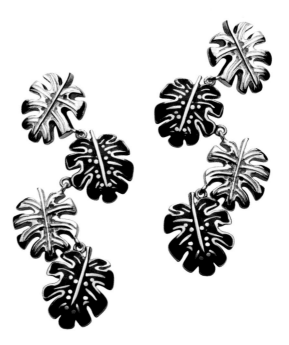

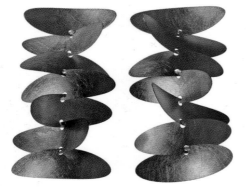

**ROC MAJORAL &
ABRIL RIBERA**
Samoa

Media: silver, gold

Photo: Majoral

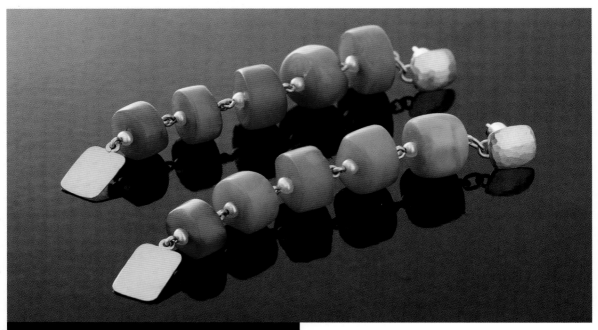

**LISA BLACK**
Tibetan Amber Drop Earrings

Media: vintage Tibetan amber beads,
pearls, 22ct gold

Photo: Flawless Imaging

**ROC MAJORAL &
ABRIL RIBERA**
Fiji

Media: gold, chrome dioxide

Photo: Majoral

**PETRA CLASS**
Big Green

Media: tourmaline, chrome diopside, peridot,
emerald, 22ct and 18ct gold

Photo: Hap Sakwa

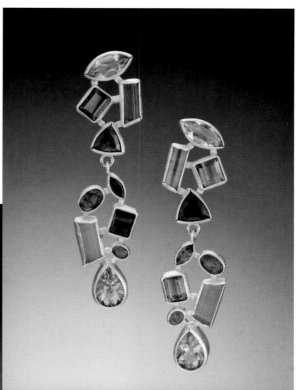

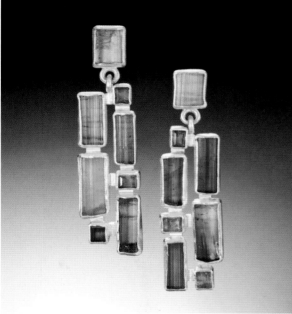

**PETRA CLASS**
Emerald Tourmaline

Media: tourmaline crystals, emeralds,
22ct and 18ct gold

Photo: Hap Sakwa

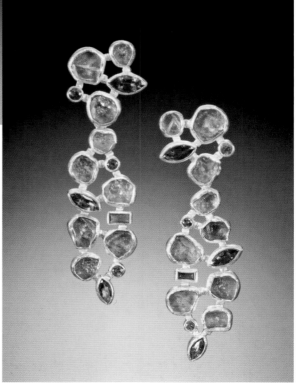

**PETRA CLASS**
Sapphire Dangles

Media: sapphire, uncut sapphire,
22ct and 18ct gold

Photo: Hap Sakwa

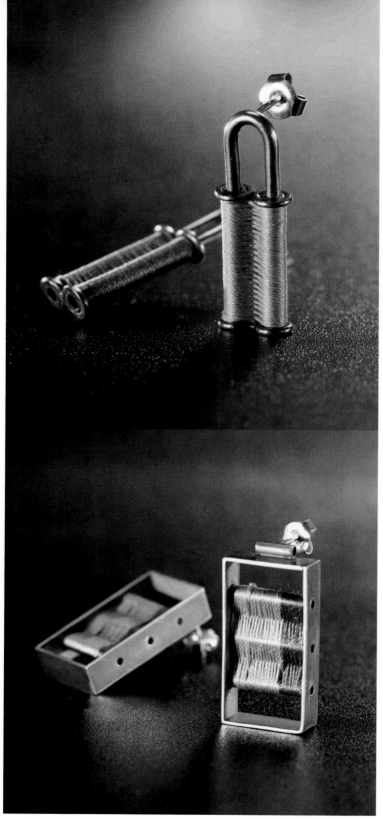

**MARIANA VISO ROJAS**
Twin

Media: silver, silk thread

Photo: Rafael Tirado

**MARIANA VISO ROJAS**
Loom

Media: silver, silk thread

Photo: Rafael Tirado

**PAULA ESTRADA**
Winged – Flies Series

Medium: 925 silver

Photo: Rafael Tirado

**PAULA ESTRADA**
Metamorphosis of the Scarab –
Insects Series

Medium: 925 silver

Photo: Rafael Tirado

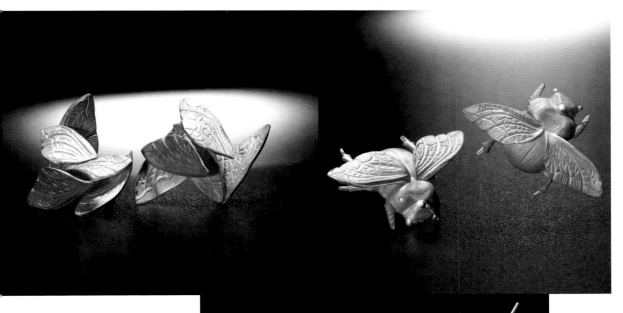

**PAULA ESTRADA**
Single Wings – Flies Series

Medium: 925 silver

Photo: Rafael Tirado

**LUÍS MÉNDEZ ARTESANOS**
Seeded Buttons

Media: 18ct yellow gold, natural ruby

Photo: Luís F. Lorenzo

**LUÍS MÉNDEZ ARTESANOS**
Horseshoe Earrings

Medium: 18ct yellow gold

Photo: Luís F. Lorenzo

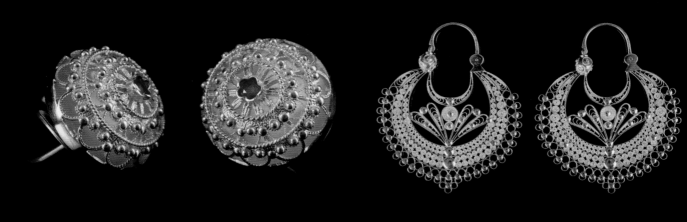

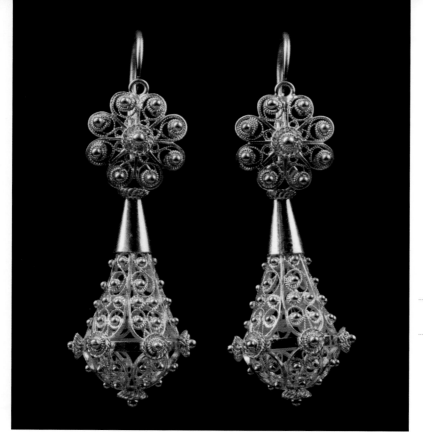

**LUÍS MÉNDEZ ARTESANOS**
Pear Earrings

Medium: 18ct yellow gold

Photo: Luís F. Lorenzo

**LUÍS MÉNDEZ ARTESANOS**
Galapagos

Medium: 18ct yellow gold

Photo: Luís F. Lorenzo

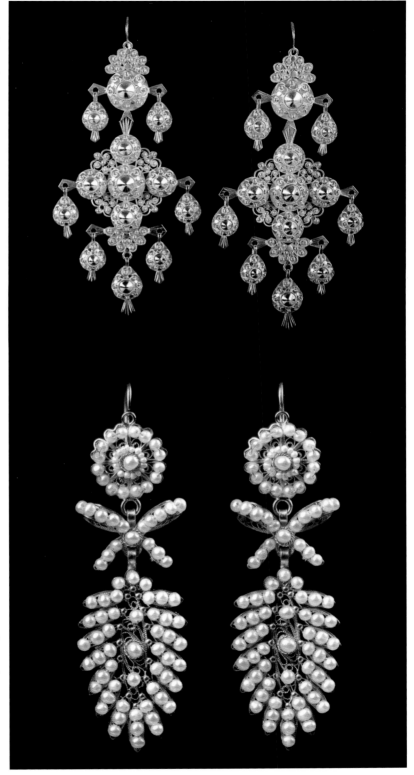

**LUÍS MÉNDEZ ARTESANOS**
Wheat Ear Earrings

Media: 18ct yellow gold, seed pearls

Photo: Luís F. Lorenzo

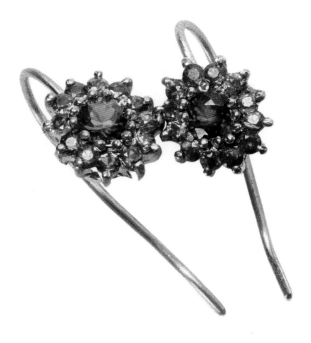

**JULIA DEVILLE**
Mourning Earrings

Media: white gold, rubies

Photo: Terence Bogue

**ANTJE STOLZ**
Stoneskins I

Media: latex, gold-plated 925 silver

Photo: Antje Stolz

**ANTJE STOLZ**
Stoneskins II

Media: latex, gold-plated 925 silver

Photo: Antje Stolz

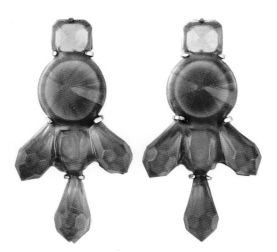

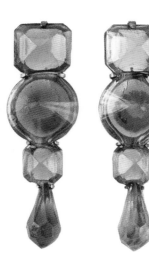

**NICOLAS ESTRADA**
Scarabs with Calla Lilies

Media: silver, pearls, mother-of-pearl,
coral

Photo: Nicolas Estrada

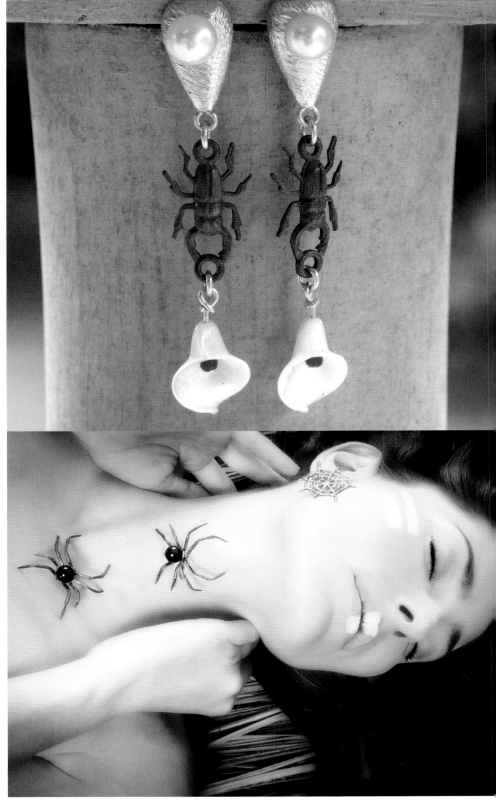

**MARTA CODERQUE**
Black Widow

Media: silver with black patina,
green aventurine

Photo: Coderque Design

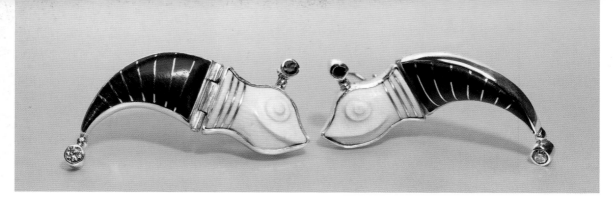

**GUNTIS LAUDERS**
Kiss

Media: 925 silver, ivory, ebony,
sapphire, zircon

Photo: Maija Muizniece

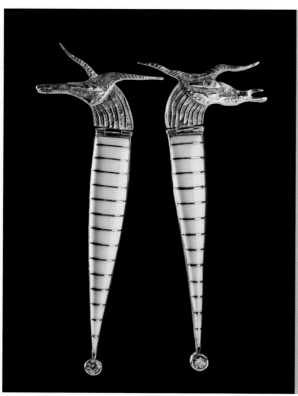

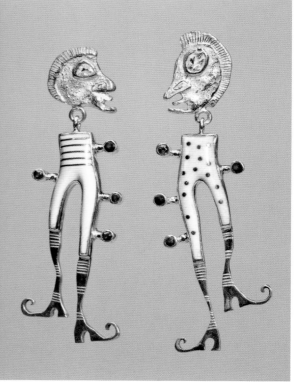

**GUNTIS LAUDERS**
Jealousy

Media: 925 silver, ivory, citrine

Photo: Maija Muizniece

**GUNTIS LAUDERS**
Dance

Media: 925 silver, ivory, garnet

Photo: Maija Muizniece

**JANIS VILKS**
Monk 2

Media: 925 silver, nephrite, onyx

Photo: Maija Muizniece

**JANIS VILKS**
Monk 1

Media: 925 silver, nephrite, onyx

Photo: Maija Muizniece

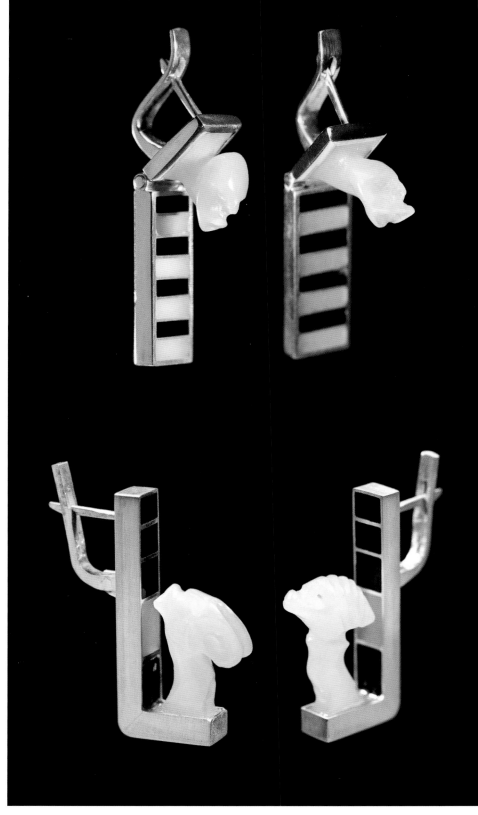

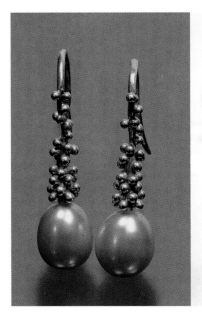

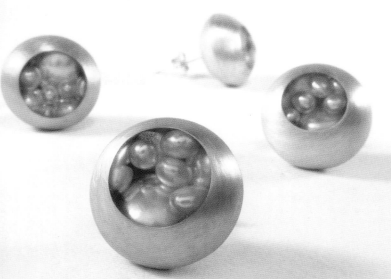

**SOPHIA GEORGIOPOULOU**
Gold 'Old Work' Earrings

Media: 18ct gold, South Sea pearls

Photo: Sophia Georgiopoulou

**ANNIE TUNG**
Pearl Studs

Media: 18ct gold, silver, freshwater
pearls, resin

Photo: Annie Tung

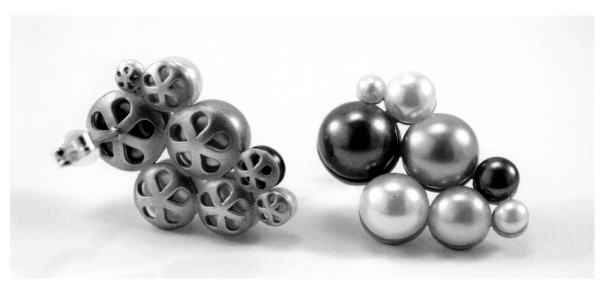

**ANNIE TUNG**
Bubbles – Pearl Studs

Media: silver, cultured freshwater
pearls

Photo: Annie Tung

**LISA BLACK**
Coral Teardrop Earrings

Media: pale coral, pearl, 22ct gold

Photo: Flawless Imaging

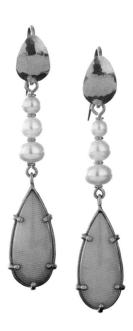

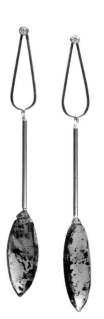

**VANESSA LEU**
Reverie Earrings

Media: kyanite, 18ct white gold

Photo: Woomin Dennis Chung

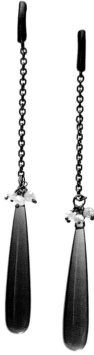

**VANESSA LEU**
Radiant Cascade Earrings with
Smoky Quartz & Rough Diamonds

Media: smoky quartz, rough diamonds,
18ct black gold

Photo: Woomin Dennis Chung

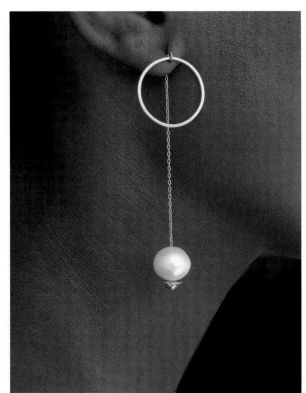

**IMMA GIBERT**
Dot and Line

Media: cultured pearl, yellow gold

Photo: Imma Gibert

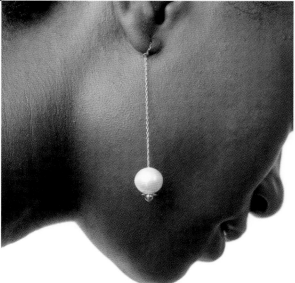

**IMMA GIBERT**
Pendulum

Media: cultured pearl, yellow gold

Photo: Imma Gibert

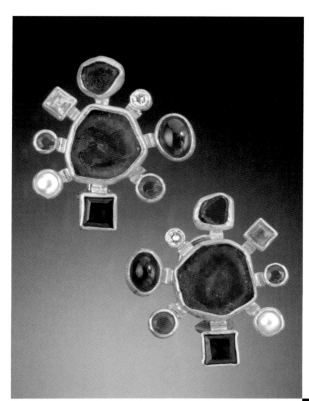

**PETRA CLASS**
Red Stars

Media: diamond, tourmaline, ruby, sapphire, pearls, 22ct and 18ct gold

Photo: Hap Sakwa

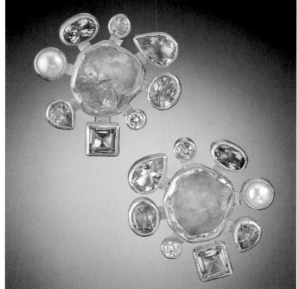

**PETRA CLASS**
Blue Yellow Stars

Media: aquamarine, diamond, topaz, citrine, pearls, 22ct and 18ct gold

Photo: Hap Sakwa

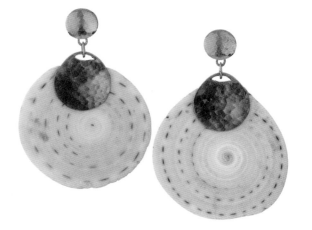

**LISA BLACK**
Papuan New Guinean Shell
Money as Earring

Media: vintage Papua New Guinean
conus shell disc, 22ct gold

Photo: Flawless Imaging

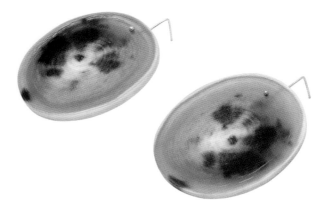

**WALKA STUDIO
(Claudia Betancourt & Nano Pulgar)**
Sacred Bull

Media: ox horn, 950 silver

Photo: Karen Clunes

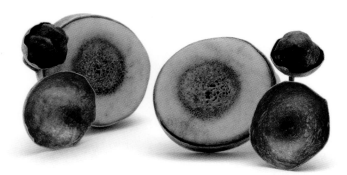

**BIBA SCHUTZ**
X's 3

Media: 925 silver, carved antler,
green jade

Photo: Ron Boszko

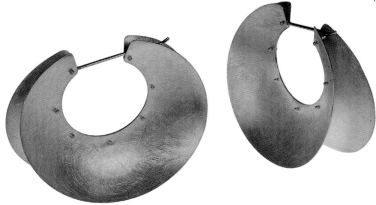

**ROC MAJORAL &
ABRIL RIBERA**
Bombay

Medium: gold

Photo: Majoral

**ELISA PAIVA**
Waves Hoop Earrings

Medium: gold-plated silver

Photo: Elisa Paiva

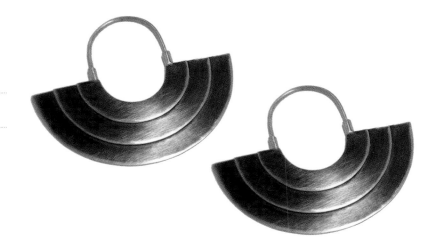

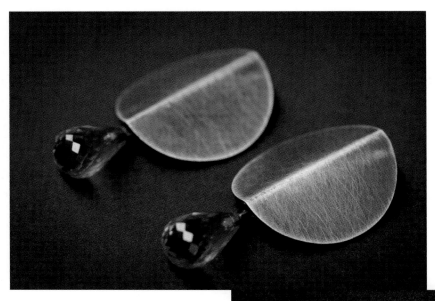

**BEATRIZ FABRES
BARAHONA**
Untitled

Media: silver, citrine quartz

Photo: Meghan Roberts

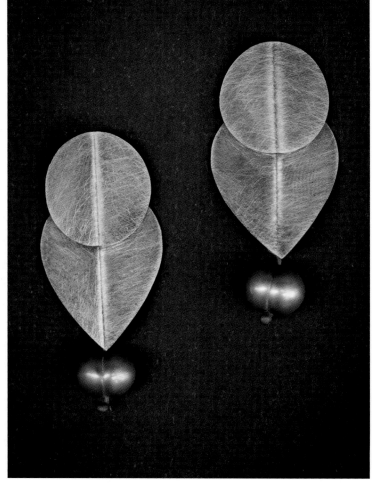

**BEATRIZ FABRES
BARAHONA**
Owl Pearls

Media: silver, river pearls

Photo: Meghan Roberts

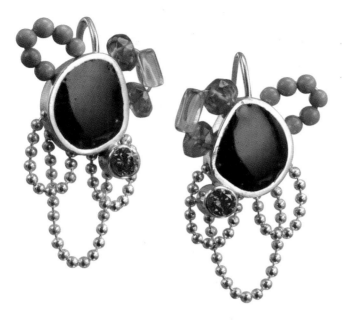

**ALEXIS KOSTUK**
Swing Earrings

Media: 925 silver, resin, cubic
zirconia, pearls, peridot

Photo: Paul Ambtman

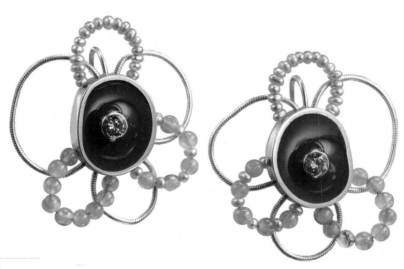

**ALEXIS KOSTUK**
Rose Earrings

Media: 925 silver, resin, cubic
zirconia, pearls, cornelian

Photo: Paul Ambtman

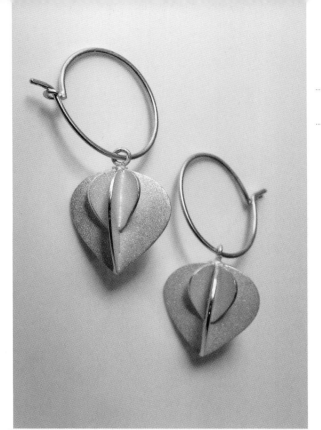

**ANA MARÍA RAMÍREZ MOURE**
Rings with Seeds

Media: 18ct gold, 925 silver

Photo: Ana María Ramírez Moure

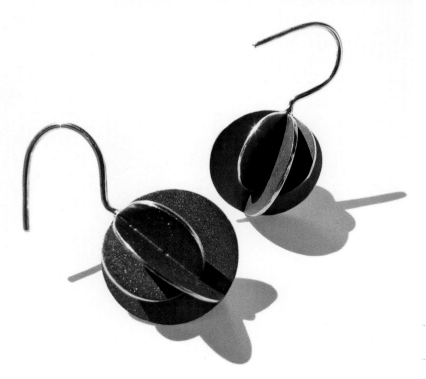

**ANA MARÍA RAMÍREZ MOURE**
Seed Pendants

Medium: 925 silver

Photo: Ana María Ramírez Moure

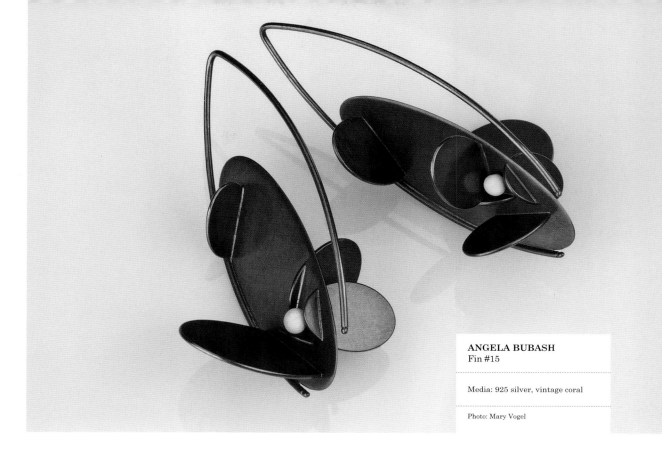

**ANGELA BUBASH**
Fin #15

Media: 925 silver, vintage coral

Photo: Mary Vogel

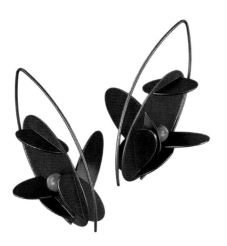

**ANGELA BUBASH**
Fin #28

Media: 925 silver, vintage coral

Photo: Mary Vogel

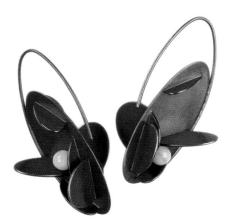

**ANGELA BUBASH**
Fin #29

Media: 925 silver, vintage coral

Photo: Mary Vogel

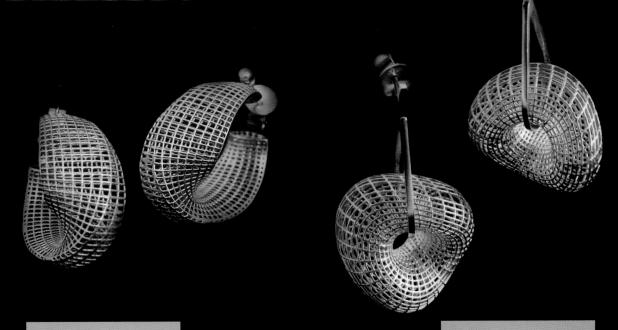

**HELLA GANOR**
Small Mobius

Medium: 14ct gold

Photo: Hella Ganor

**HELLA GANOR**
Small Twisted Torus

Medium: 14ct gold

Photo: Hella Ganor

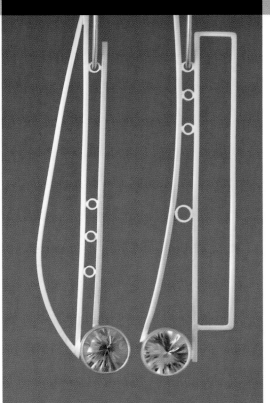

**JACKIE ANDERSON**
Linear Motion

Media: 925 silver, 10ct gold,
prasiolite

Photo: Jackie Anderson

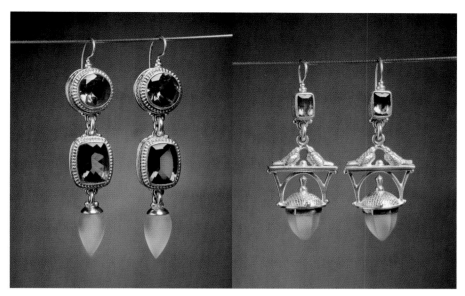

**JOHN BLAIR**
Untitled

Media: 925 silver, blue topaz,
amethyst, frosted quartz

Photo: John Dean

**JOHN BLAIR**
Bird Song

Media: 925 silver, green
tourmaline, frosted quartz

Photo: John Dean

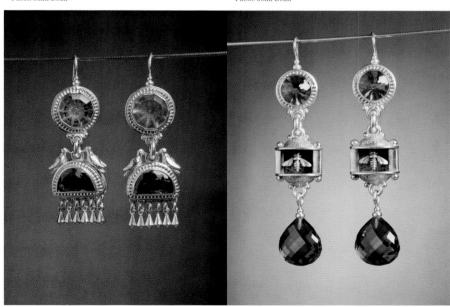

**JOHN BLAIR**
Birds

Media: 925 silver, citrine,
blue topaz

Photo: John Dean

**JOHN BLAIR**
Queen Bee

Media: 925 silver, citrine,
cognac quartz

Photo: John Dean

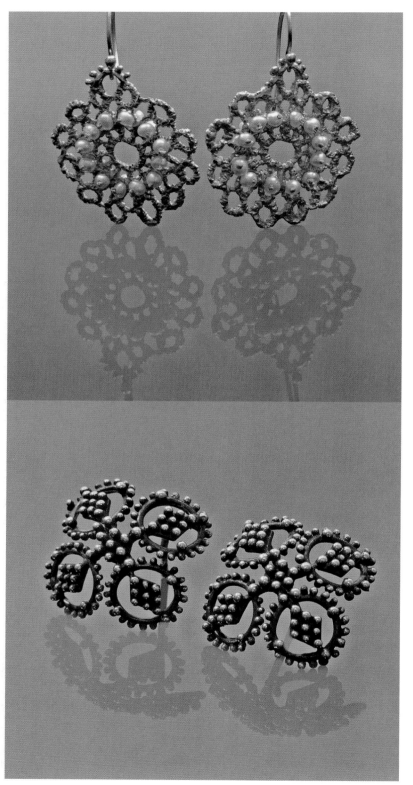

**SOPHIA GEORGIOPOULOU**
Old Lace and Lavender Silk
Earrings

Media: 18ct gold, pearls, silk

Photo: Sophia Georgiopoulou

**SOPHIA GEORGIOPOULOU**
Constantinople Domed
Earrings

Medium: 925 silver

Photo: Sophia Georgiopoulou

**KARIM OUKID OUKSEL**
Water Elements

Media: silver, natural pearl, coral

Photo: Pau Esculies

**KARIM OUKID OUKSEL**
Creole Blue

Media: silver, enamel, chalcedony

Photo: Pau Esculies

**KARIM OUKID OUKSEL**
Creole Black

Media: silver, enamel, onyx

Photo: Joan Soto

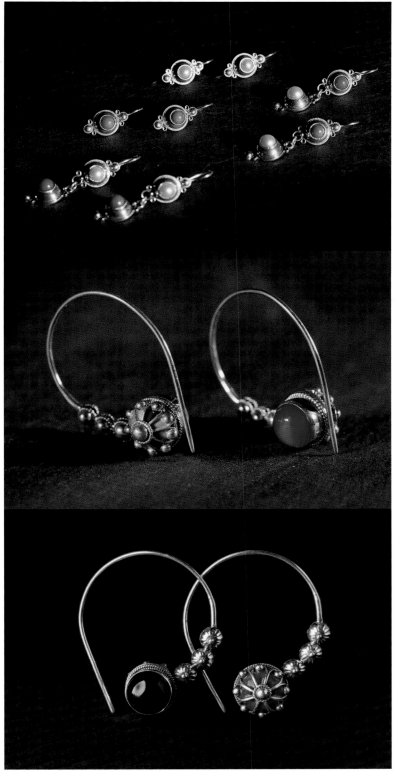

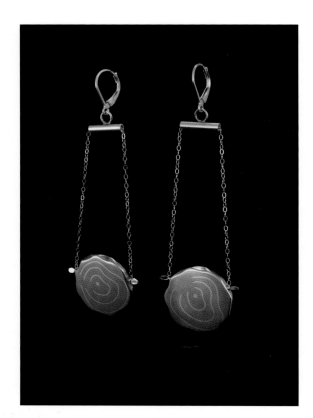

**J. ADRIANNE DIENNO**
Trapeze Tree Rings

Media: nickel, silver, brass

Photo: Dustin Dienno

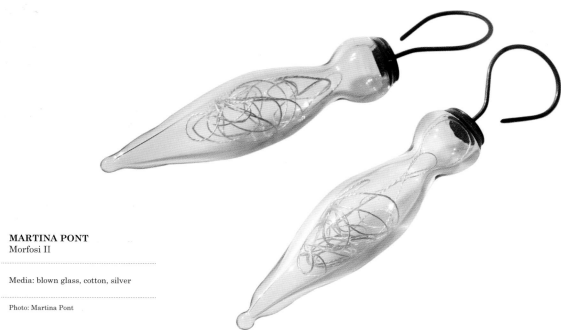

**MARTINA PONT**
Morfosi II

Media: blown glass, cotton, silver

Photo: Martina Pont

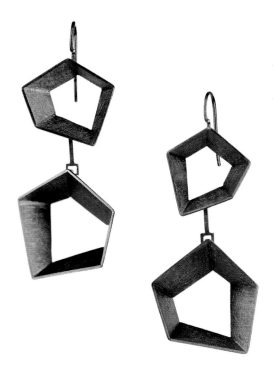

**BABETTE VON DOHNANYI**
Open Space

Medium: 925 silver

Photo: Federico Cavicchioli

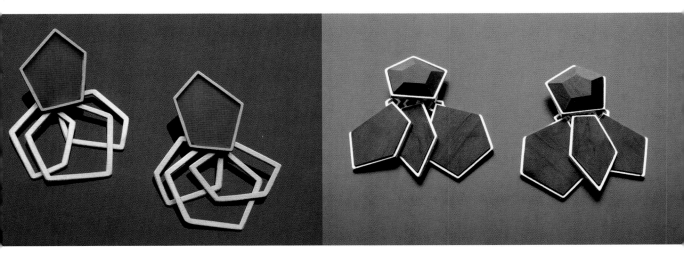

**BABETTE VON DOHNANYI**
Polyps

Media: 925 silver, blue PMMA

Photo: Federico Cavicchioli

**BABETTE VON DOHNANYI**
Polyps

Media: 925 silver, jet

Photo: Federico Cavicchioli

**DAMIÀ MULET**
Portal des Celler

Media: silver, Santanyí stone

Photo: Jaume Segura Moragues

**DAMIÀ MULET**
Portal de Sa Salera

Media: silver, Santanyí stone

Photo: Jaume Segura Moragues

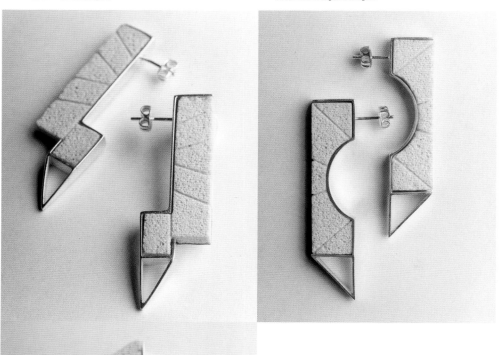

**DAMIÀ MULET**
Portal de Sa Portassa

Media: silver, Santanyí stone

Photo: Jaume Segura Moragues

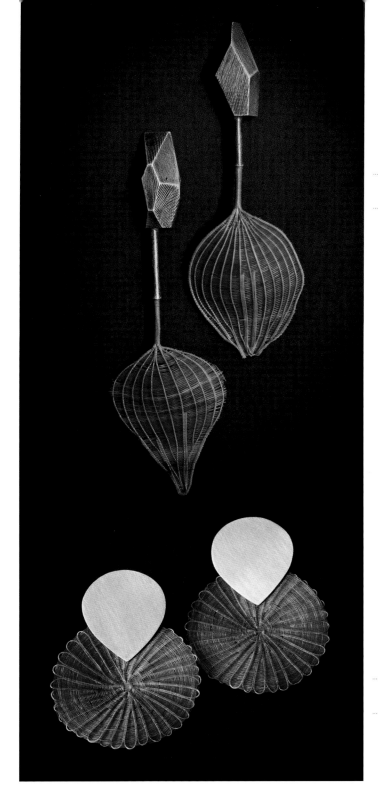

**BEATRIZ FABRES
BARAHONA**
Leaves

Media: silver, dyed horsehair

Photo: Meghan Roberts

**BEATRIZ FABRES
BARAHONA**
Fan Earrings

Media: openwork silver, horsehair

Photo: Gennaro Navarra

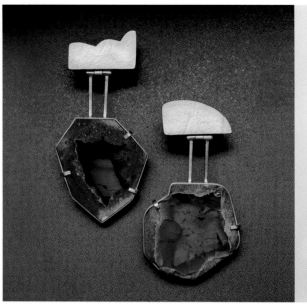

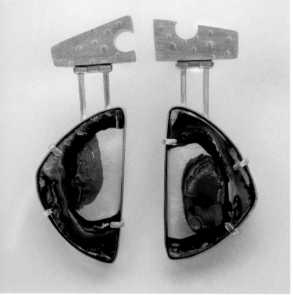

**BARBARA CHRISTIE**
GH 28458

Media: 18ct yellow gold, hinged textured
boxes with claw-set fire opal crystals

Photo: Barbara Christie

**BARBARA CHRISTIE**
GH 32272

Media: 18ct yellow gold, hinged textured gold
boxes with boulder opal crystals

Photo: Barbara Christie

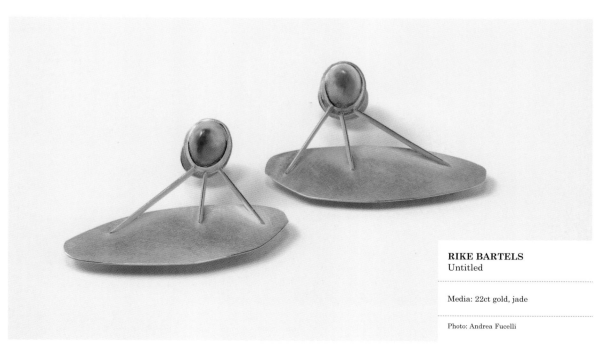

**RIKE BARTELS**
Untitled

Media: 22ct gold, jade

Photo: Andrea Fucelli

**VIKKI KASSIORAS**
Hades

Media: 18ct yellow gold, onyx, rubies

Photo: Terence Bogue

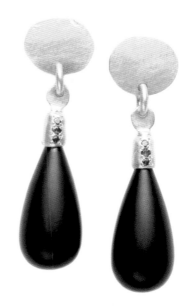

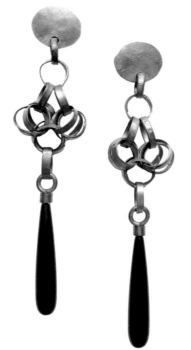

**VIKKI KASSIORAS**
Untitled

Media: 925 silver, onyx

Photo: Terence Bogue

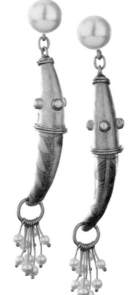

**LISA BLACK**
Carved PNG Tooth Earrings

Media: Papua New Guinean canine
teeth, 22ct gold, pearl

Photo: Flawless Imaging

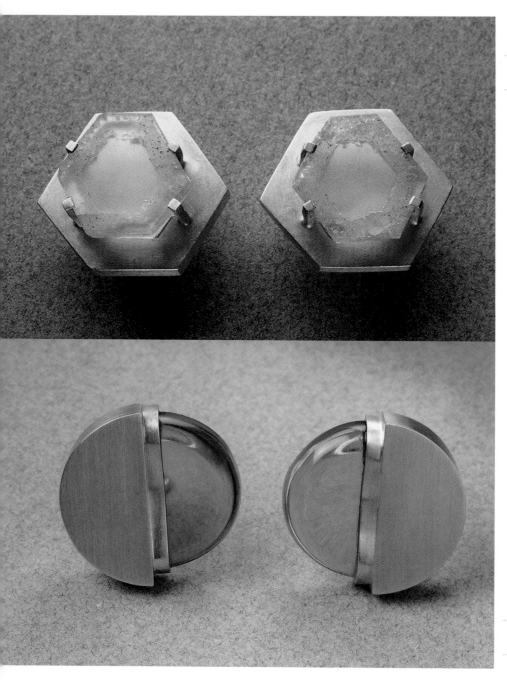

**PILAR GARRIGOSA**
Untitled

Media: 18ct gold, aquamarines

Photo: Nos y Soto

**PILAR GARRIGOSA**
Untitled

Media: 18ct gold, amber

Photo: Nos y Soto

**CARMEN PINTOR – GALERÍA**
**MEKO JOYERÍA DE AUTOR**
Stone

Media: 18ct gold, amethyst

Photo: Carmen Pintor

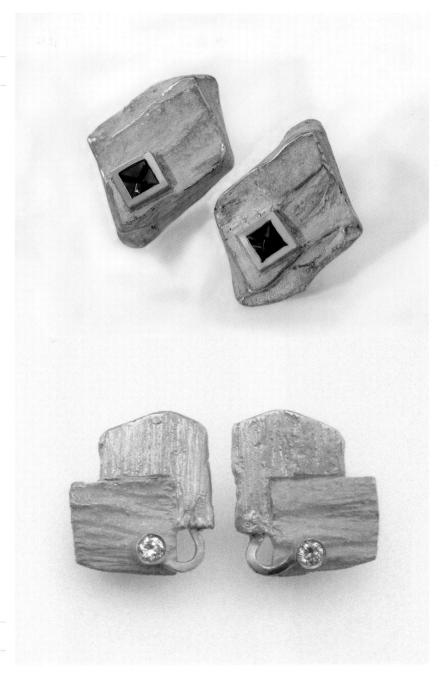

**CARMEN PINTOR – GALERÍA**
**MEKO JOYERÍA DE AUTOR**
Haiku

Media: 18ct gold, diamonds

Photo: Carmen Pintor

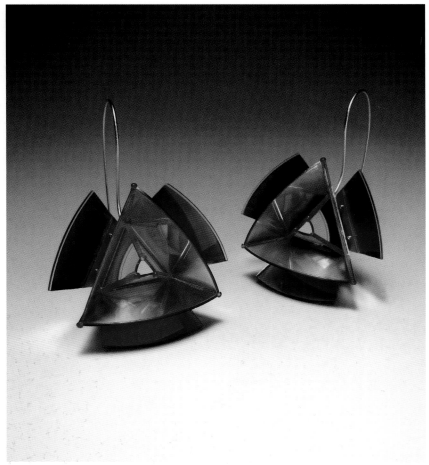

**CHUN-LUNG HSIEH**
Value of Light

Media: compact disc, brass,
screw, plastic

Photo: Chun-Lung Hsieh

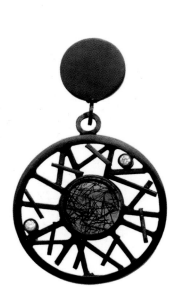 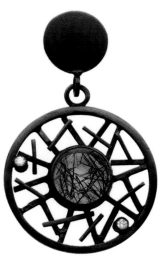

**DAPHNE KRINOS**
Earrings

Media: silver, tourmaline quartz,
diamonds

Photo: Joel Degen

**BARBARA CHRISTIE**
GH 38502

Media: 18ct yellow gold, gold boxes, onyx stones,
champagne diamond, clear diamonds

Photo: Barbara Christie

**BARBARA CHRISTIE**
GH 40145

Media: 18ct yellow gold, gold boxes, onyx
stones, coral

Photo: Barbara Christie

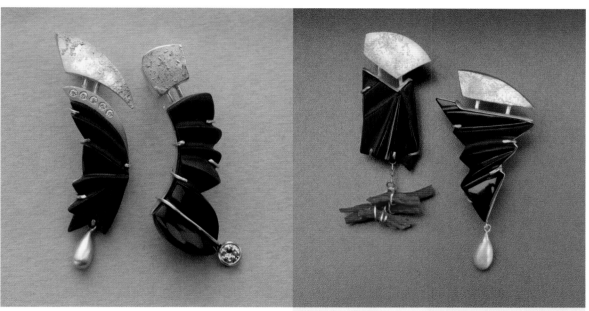

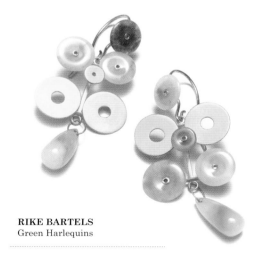

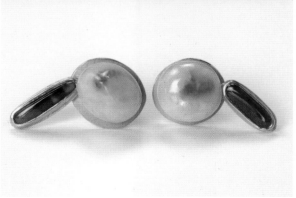

**RIKE BARTELS**
Green Harlequins

Media: 22ct gold, jade

Photo: Jens Mauritz

**RIKE BARTELS**
Ducks

Media: 22ct gold, jade

Photo: Andrea Fucelli

**RIKE BARTELS**
Ear Pad

........................................

Media: 22ct gold, slate

........................................

Photo: Jens Mauritz

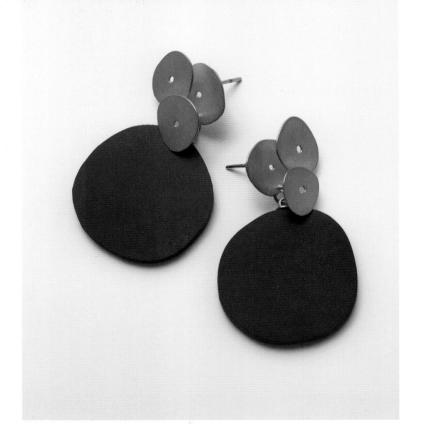

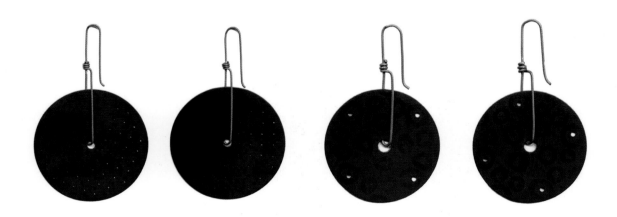

**TORE SVENSSON**
Untitled

........................................

Media: steel, titanium

........................................

Photo: Franz Karl

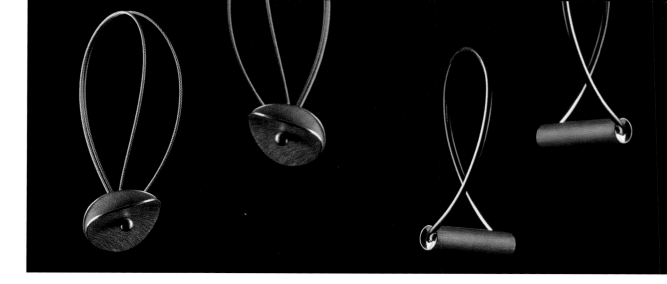

**SALVADOR MALLOL**
Sash

Media: silver, steel

Photo: Lafotografica

**SALVADOR MALLOL**
Gold Figure-of-8 Earrings

Media: yellow gold, white gold

Photo: Lafotografica

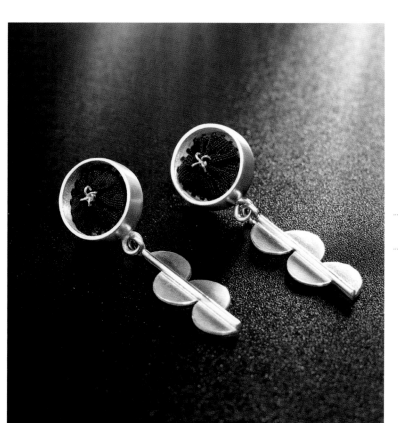

**MARIANA VISO ROJAS**
Laila

Media: silver, fabric

Photo: Rafael Tirado

**MAREEN ALBURG DUNCKER**
Half Lemons

Media: silver, peridot

Photo: Udo W. Beier

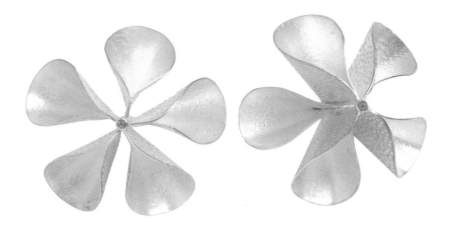

**MARTA SÀNCHEZ OMS**
Ophelia

Media: silver, rough green and pink
tourmalines

Photo: Marta Sànchez Oms

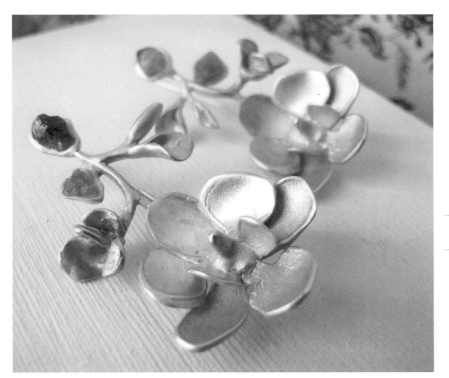

**CARLES SERRANO – DELAJOIA**
Antiqua I

Media: silver, 18ct green gold, cultured
pearls

Photo: Carles Serrano

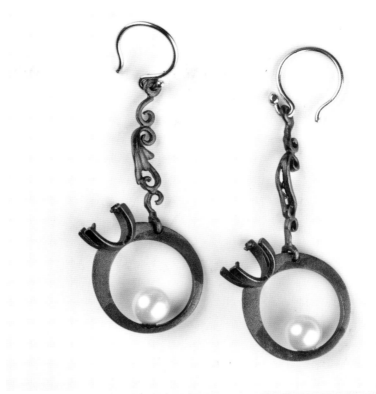

**CARLES SERRANO – DELAJOIA**
Antiqua V

Media: silver, 18ct green gold, cultured
pearls

Photo: Carles Serrano

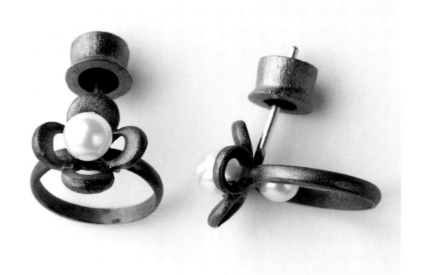

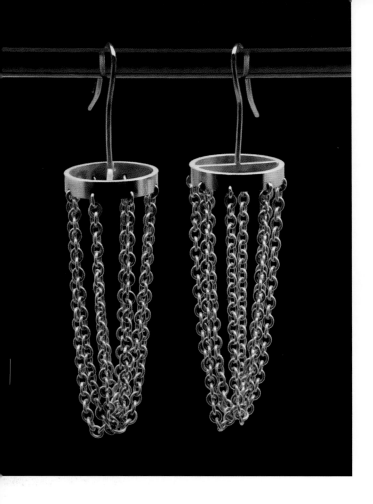

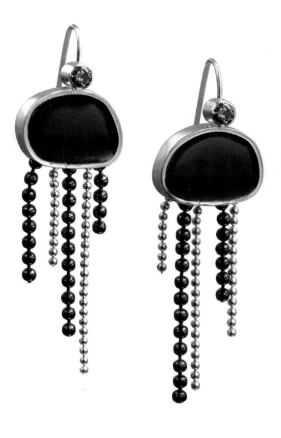

**EMILY WATSON**
Maypole Earrings

Medium: 925 silver

Photo: Emily Watson

**ALEXIS KOSTUK**
Rain Earrings

Media: 925 silver, steel, resin,
cubic zirconia

Photo: Paul Ambtman

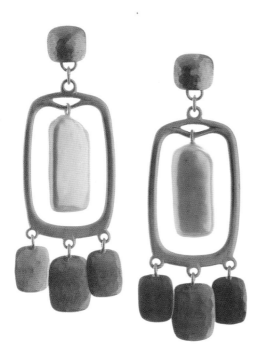

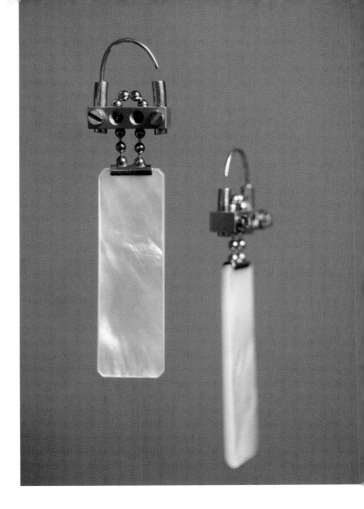

**LISA BLACK**
Freshwater Pearl Chandelier
Drop Earrings

Media: freshwater pearls, 22ct gold

Photo: Flawless Imaging

**ISABELLE FUSTINONI**
Casino

Media: bronze, steel, mother-of-pearl

Photo: Wonder*dim

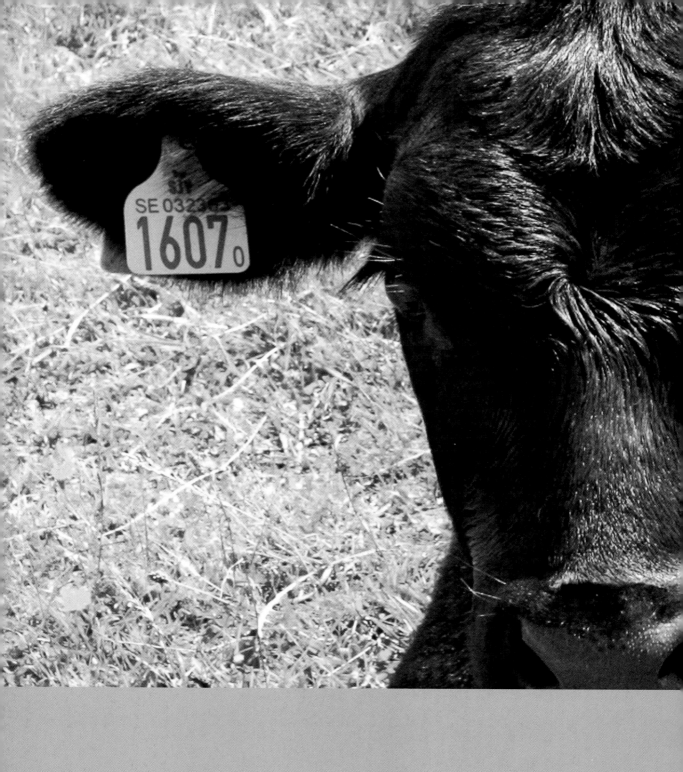

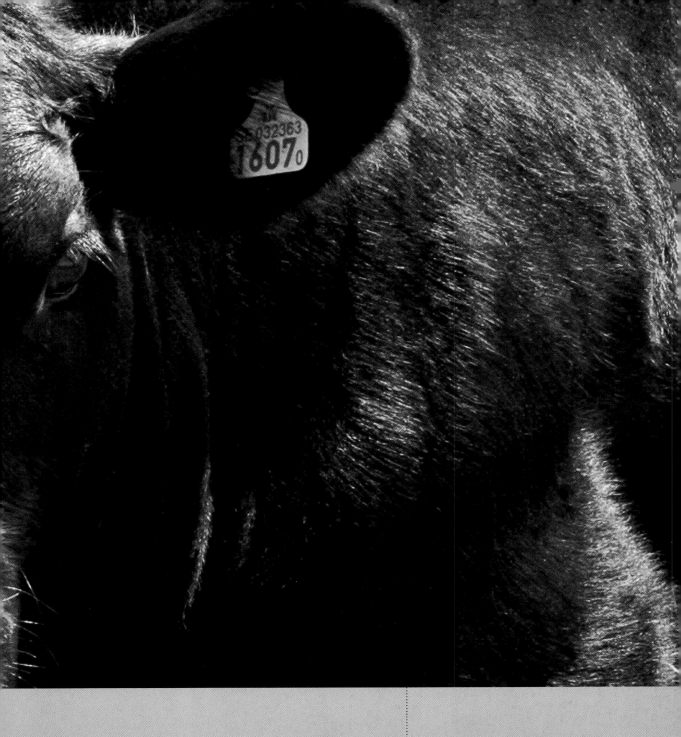

DARING

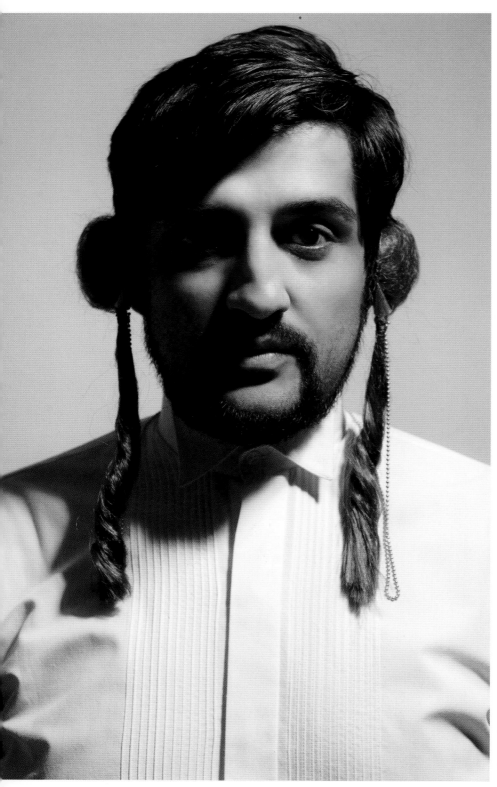

**RODRIGO ACOSTA ARIAS**
The Permissiveness of your God

Media: earrings, hair, silver, brass

Photo: Adolfo López

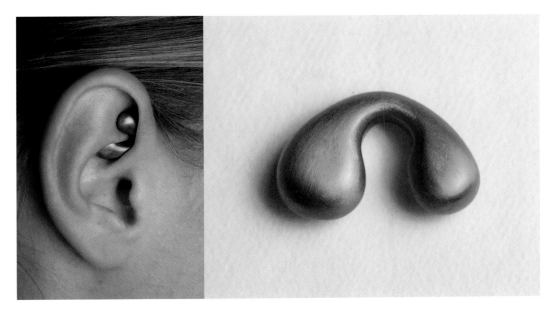

**LILI ZSABOKORSZKY**
Without Hole

Medium: aluminium

Photo: Apor Püspöki

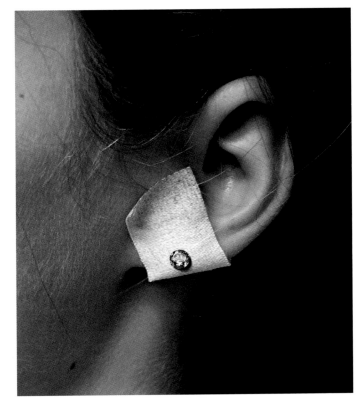

**MARTIN PAPCÚN**
Earring

Media: sticking plaster, aquamarine

Photo: Martin Papcún

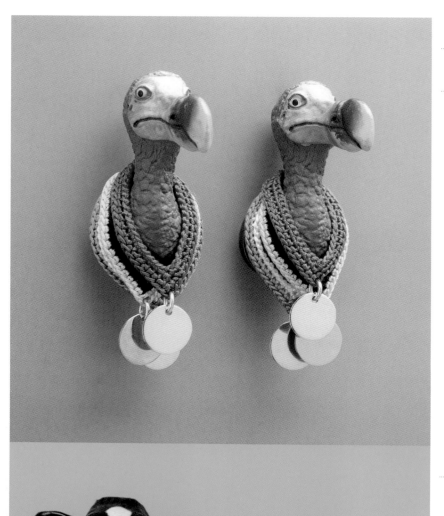

**FELIEKE VAN DER LEEST**
The Outsiders

Media: yellow, white and red gold, plastic animals, textile, silver

Photo: Eddo Hartmann

**FELIEKE VAN DER LEEST**
The Kalf Sisters

Media: plastic animals, silver, gold, plastic pearls, cubic zirconia

Photo: Eddo Hartmann

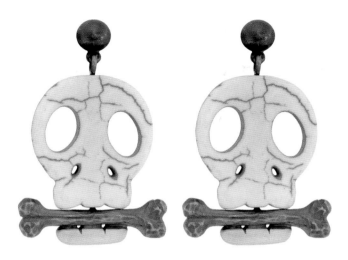

**MARTA CODERQUE**
Flat Skull

Media: silver, howlite skull

Photo: Coderque Design

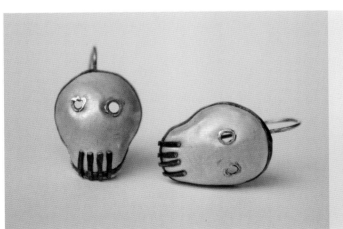

**SOPHIE BOUDUBAN**
Head

Media: iron, silver

Photo: Sophie Bouduban

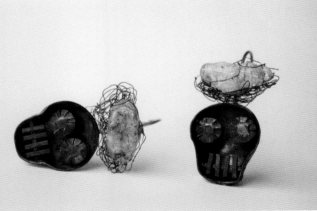

**SOPHIE BOUDUBAN**
Cloud

Media: iron, glass

Photo: Sophie Bouduban

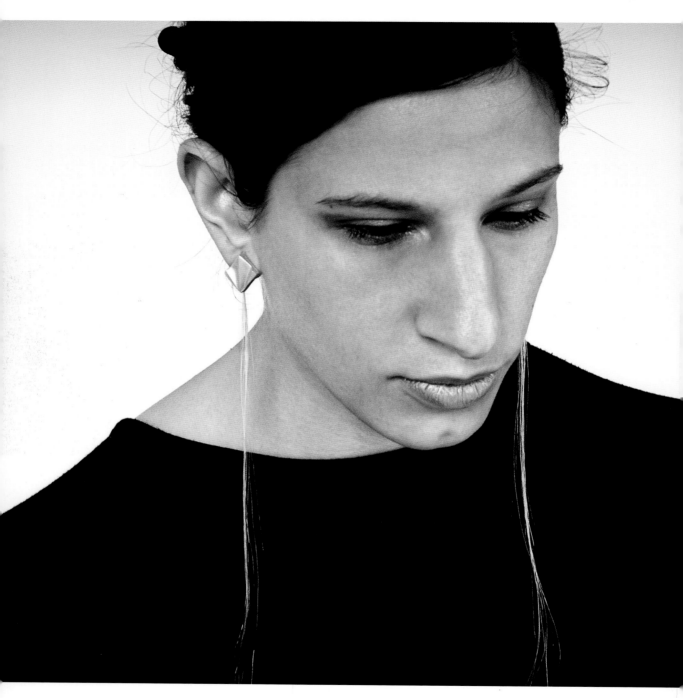

**EVA BURTON**
Kites

Media: silver, horsehair

Photo: Eva Burton

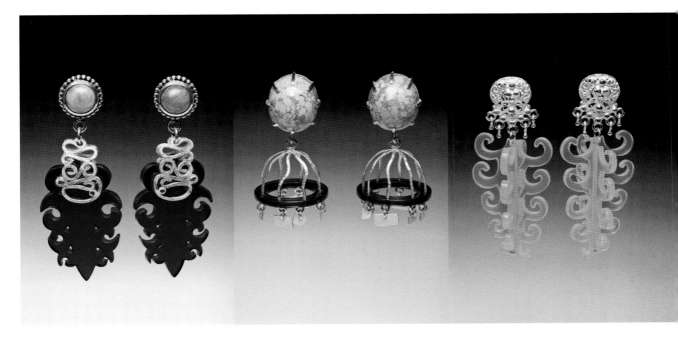

**JOSÉE DESJARDINS**
A Jeweller's Travel
Memorabilia: Bollywood 7

Media: 925 silver, PMMA,
aquamarine

Photo: Anthony McLean

**JOSÉE DESJARDINS**
A Jeweller's Travel
Memorabilia: Prem Muna 4

Media: 925 silver, PMMA, turquoise

Photo: Anthony McLean

**JOSÉE DESJARDINS**
A Jeweller's Travel
Memorabilia: Bollywood 5

Media: 925 silver, PMMA

Photo: Anthony McLean

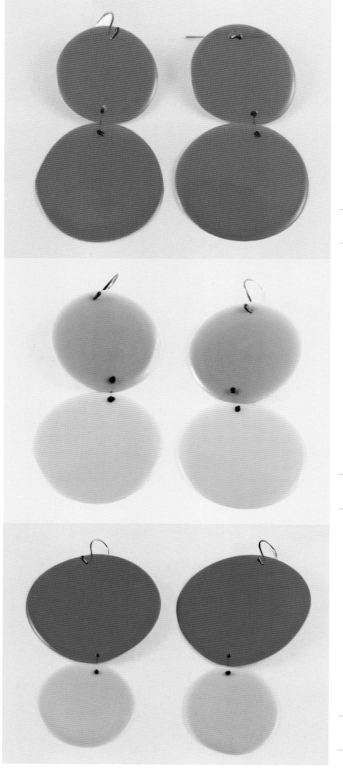

**ELA BAUER**
Untitled

Media: plastic, silver

Photo: Ela Bauer

**ELA BAUER**
Untitled

Media: plastic, silver

Photo: Ela Bauer

**ELA BAUER**
Untitled

Media: plastic, silver

Photo: Ela Bauer

**JULIA DEVILLE**
Calvinism Rosary Earrings

Media: silver, black rhodium plate,
black garnet

Photo: Terence Bogue

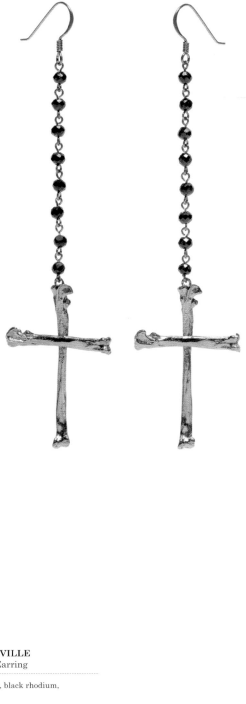

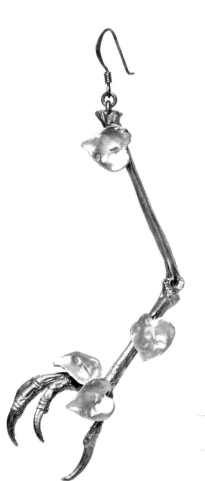

**JULIA DEVILLE**
Lily Claw Earring

Media: silver, black rhodium,
gold plate

Photo: Terence Bogue

**MIRLA FERNANDES**
Longing for the Body Series

Medium: latex with pigment

Photo: André Penteado

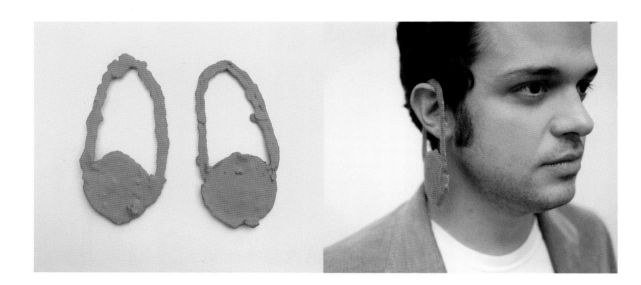

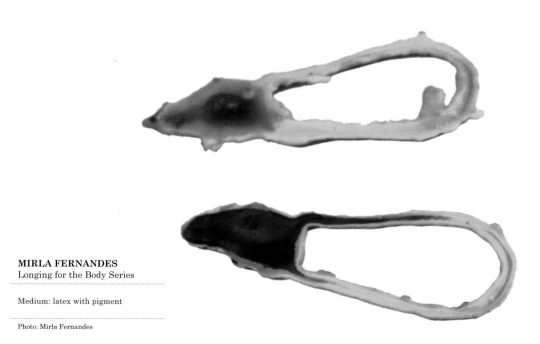

**MIRLA FERNANDES**
Longing for the Body Series

Medium: latex with pigment

Photo: Mirla Fernandes

**LOURDES CARMELO**
Saint Patience

Media: earwires, glass beads

Photo: Lourdes Carmelo & Raul Torrent

**VANESSA LEU**
Radiant Cascade Earrings
with Ethiopian Opals

Media: Ethiopian opals,
18ct black gold

Photo: Woomin Dennis Chung

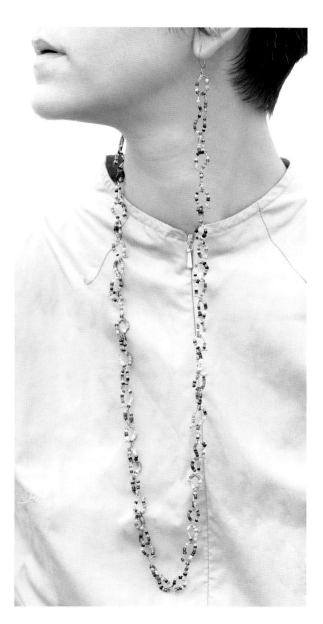

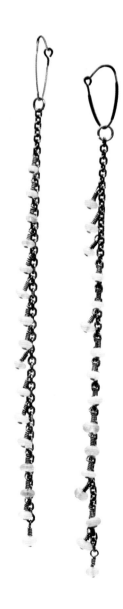

**AMY TAVERN**
Earrings

..............................................

Media: 925 silver, spray paint

..............................................

Photo: Hank Drew

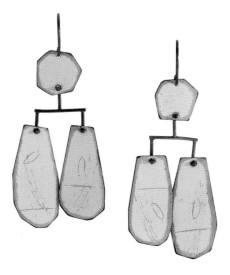

**AMY TAVERN**
Red and White Earrings

..............................................

Media: 925 silver, spray paint

..............................................

Photo: Hank Drew

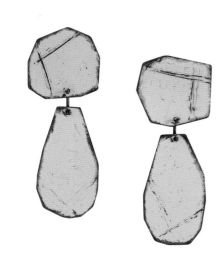

**FANNY AGNIER**
Drops 3

..............................................

Media: gold, silver, enamel

..............................................

Photo: Fanny Agnier

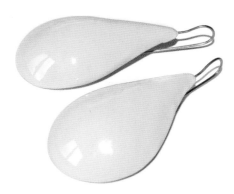

**AMY TAVERN**
Red and White Earrings

..............................................

Media: 925 silver, spray paint

..............................................

Photo: Hank Drew

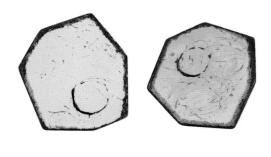

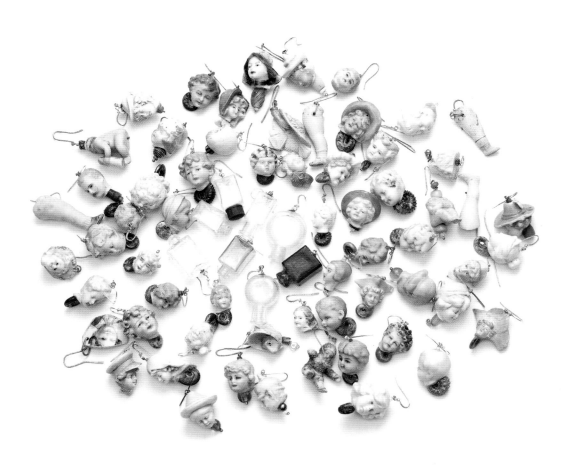

**TANIA SKLYAR**
Porcelain Laughter

Media: silver, fragments of antique
porcelain figurines

Photo: Tania Sklyar

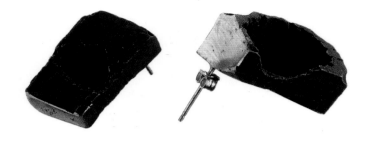

**CATALINA BRENES**
For Her

Media: silver, shibuichi

Photo: Federico Cavicchio

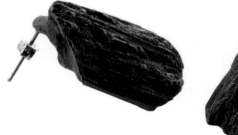 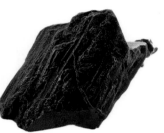

**CATALINA BRENES**
Resist

Media: silver, shibuichi

Photo: Federico Cavicchio

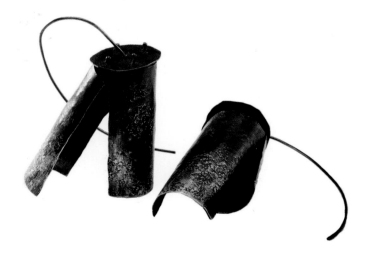

**BIBA SCHUTZ**
Towers

Medium: 925 silver

Photo: Ron Boszko

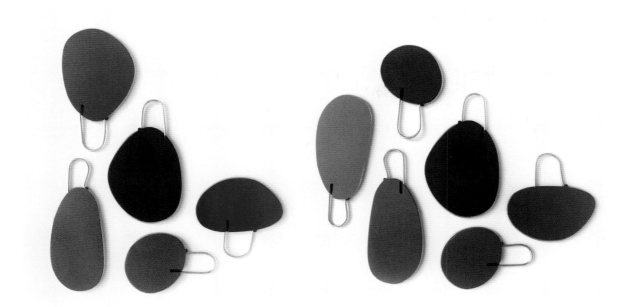

**IRIS SAAR ISAACS**
Pebble Small / Medium /
Large / Long

Media: anodized aluminium,
925 silver

Photo: Iris Saar Isaacs

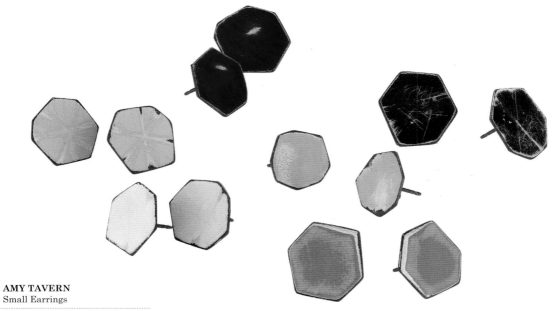

**AMY TAVERN**
Small Earrings

Media: 925 silver, spray paint

Photo: Hank Drew

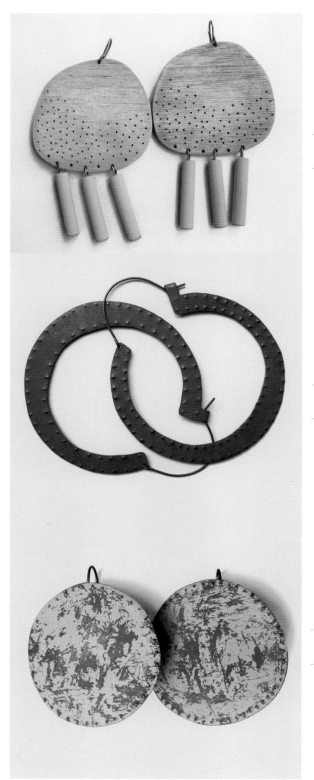

**NATALIA MILOSZ-PIEKARSKA**
Chandelier

Media: wood, 925 silver, paint

Photo: Natalia Milosz-Piekarska

**NATALIA MILOSZ-PIEKARSKA**
Mami

Media: 925 silver, paint

Photo: Natalia Milosz-Piekarska

**NATALIA MILOSZ-PIEKARSKA**
Luna

Media: 925 silver, paint

Photo: Natalia Milosz-Piekarska

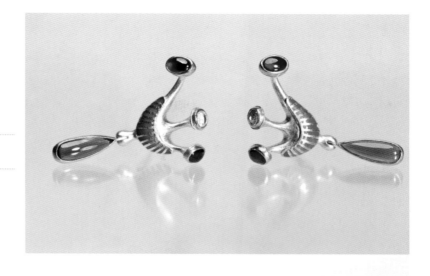

**VALDIS BROZE**
Garnet Fork

Media: 925 silver, 18ct gold, enamel, garnet

Photo: Maija Muizniece

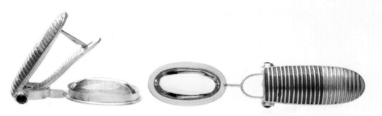

**VALDIS BROZE**
Big Bug

Media: 925 silver, enamel, topaz

Photo: Maija Muizniece

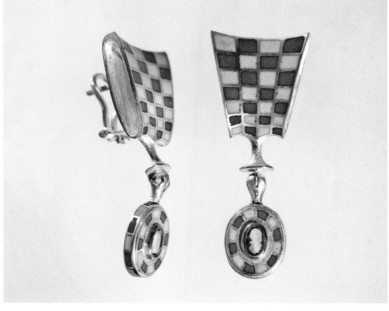

**VALDIS BROZE**
Smart Earcatcher

Media: 925 silver, 18ct gold, enamel, topaz

Photo: Maija Muizniece

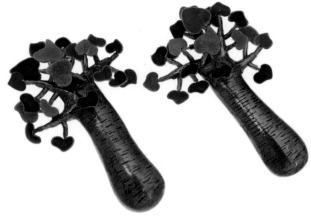

**ADRIANA HENAO MEJÍA**
Baobab – Arbórea

Media: 950 silver, glazed enamel

Photo: Jorge Mario Múnera

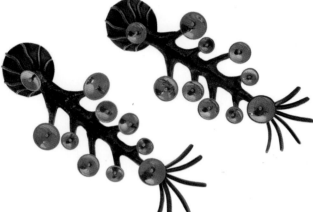

**ADRIANA HENAO MEJÍA**
The Upside-Down Tree – Arbórea

Media: 950 silver, 18ct ecological gold

Photo: Jorge Mario Múnera

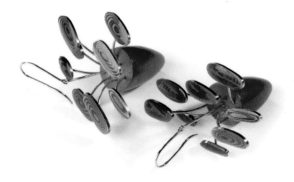

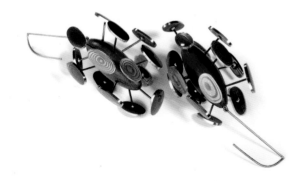

**ANGELO VERGA**
Sintered Nature 2 – Mushrooms and Flowers

Media: sintered steel, mokume gane, red gold,
enamel, wood

Photo: Beppe Bisceglia

**ANGELO VERGA**
Sintered Nature 3 – Mushrooms and Flowers

Media: sintered steel, mokume gane, titanium,
white gold, wood

Photo: Beppe Bisceglia

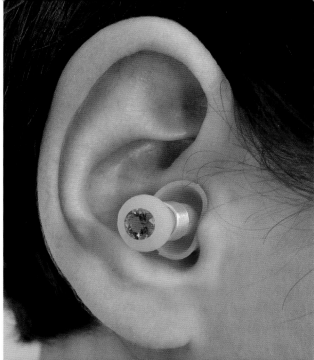

**ANDRA OANA LUPU**
Ear Plug Earrings

Media: silicone rubber ear plug,
925 silver, cubic zirconia

Photo: Andra Oana Lupu

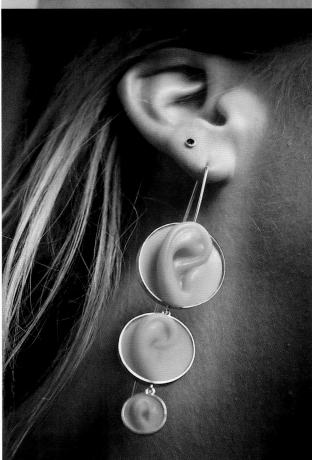

**FRÉDÉRIQUE COOMANS**
Resurrection – All Ears

Media: silver, recycled doll parts

Photo: Anne-Lise Chopin

**AMY TAVERN**
Light Blue Earrings

Media: 925 silver, spray paint

Photo: Hank Drew

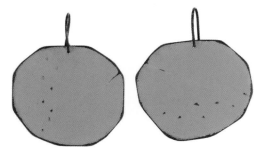

**FANNY AGNIER**
Drops 5

Media: gold, silver, enamel

Photo: Fanny Agnier

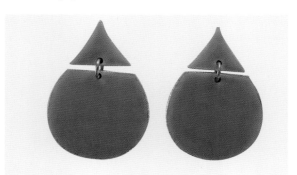

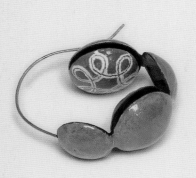

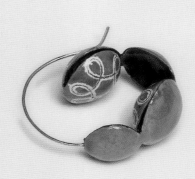

**BEATE KLOCKMANN**
Untitled

Media: iron, enamel

Photo: Beate Klockmann

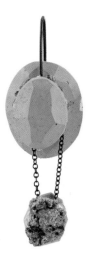

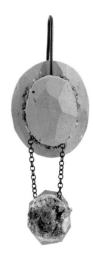

**ANTJE STOLZ**
La Fée Verte

Media: plastic, pigment, 925 silver

Photo: Antje Stolz

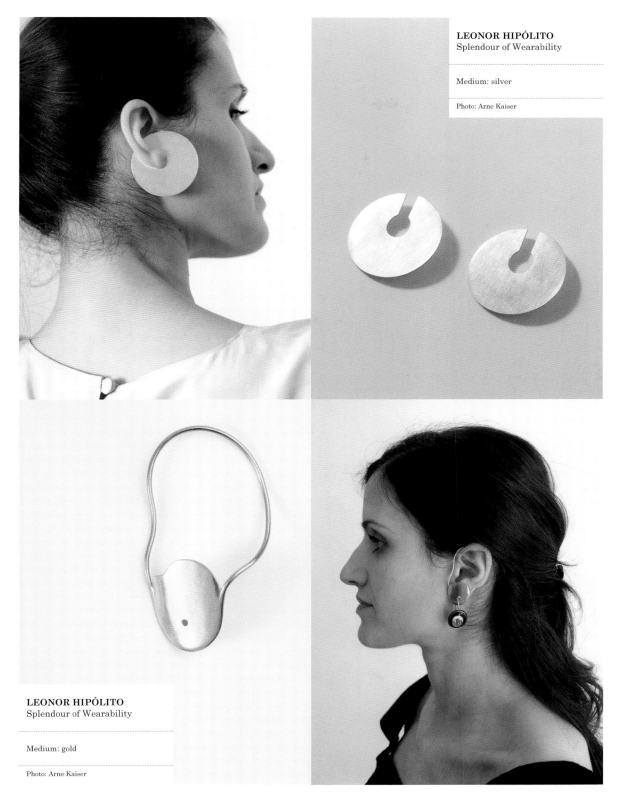

**LEONOR HIPÓLITO**
Splendour of Wearability

Medium: silver

Photo: Arne Kaiser

**LEONOR HIPÓLITO**
Splendour of Wearability

Medium: gold

Photo: Arne Kaiser

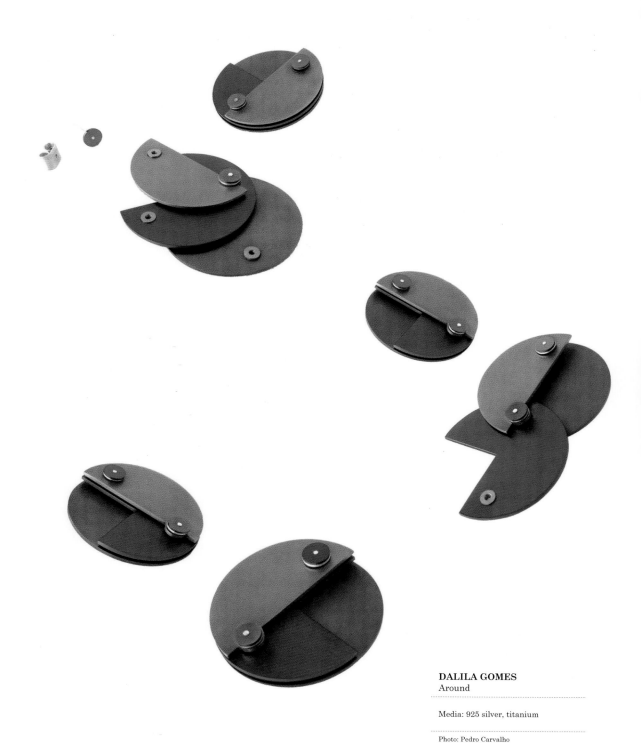

**DALILA GOMES**
Around

Media: 925 silver, titanium

Photo: Pedro Carvalho

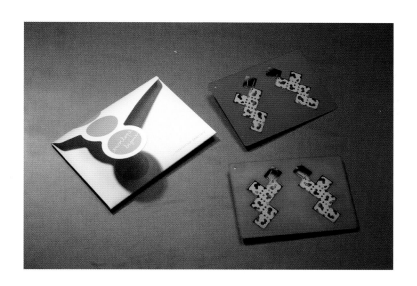

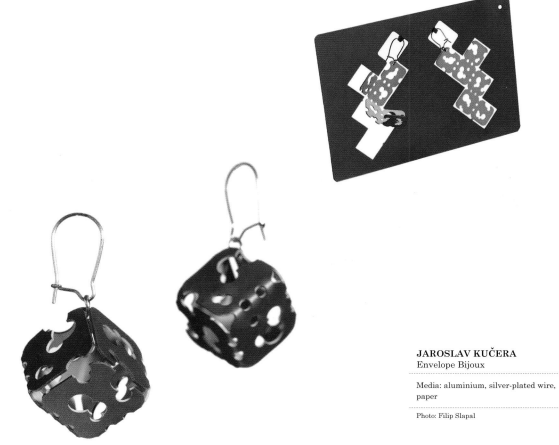

**JAROSLAV KUČERA**
Envelope Bijoux

Media: aluminium, silver-plated wire, paper

Photo: Filip Slapal

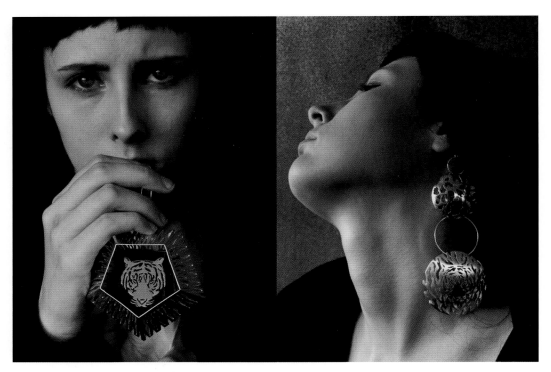

**ESTER FAIMAN**
Beyond the Era – Tiger

Media: silver, gold-plated silver,
palm wood

Photo: Ester Faiman

**ESTER FAIMAN**
Beyond the Era – Lynx

Medium: silver

Photo: Ester Faiman

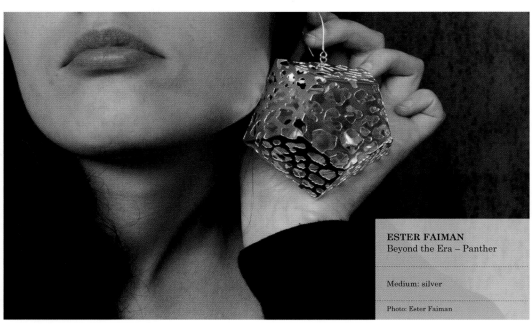

**ESTER FAIMAN**
Beyond the Era – Panther

Medium: silver

Photo: Ester Faiman

**MAREEN ALBURG DUNCKER**
Yellow Lemons

Media: lemons, silver, paint

Photo: Udo W. Beier

**BEATE KLOCKMANN**
Pair of Mountains

Media: gold, copper, enamel

Photo: Beate Klockmann

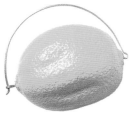
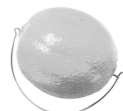
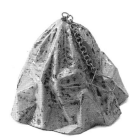
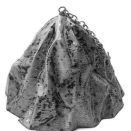

**LISA M. JOHNSON**
On the Move Series

Media: 925 silver, rose quartz, porcelain

Photo: Chandra De Buse

**TOVE KNUTS**
Molluscamolecule

Media: wooden balls, paint, silver

Photo: Tove Knuts

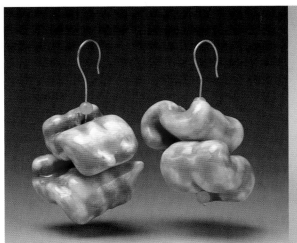
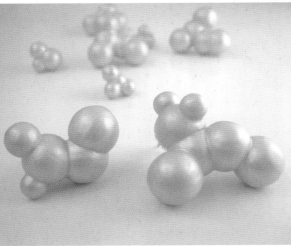

**MARLENE BEYER**
Clips

Media: natural rubber, silver

Photo: Melanie Zanin

**JENNACA DAVIES**
Lady Earrings

Medium: 925 silver

Photo: Steffen Knudsen Allen

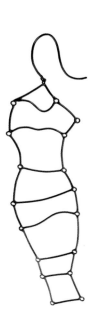

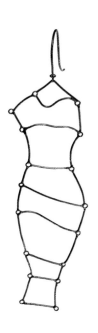

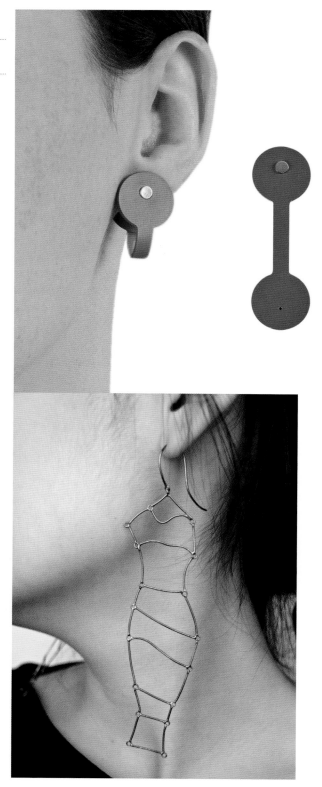

**MARÍA LILIANA RUIZ**
Floating Planet

Media: 925 silver, porcelain, floss

Photo: Lirú

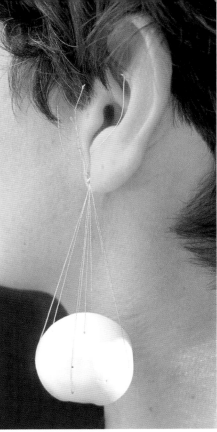

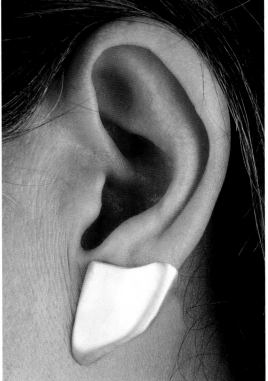

**ISA DUARTE RIBEIRO**
The Bottom of My Ears

Medium: 925 silver

Photo: Fabrice Ziegler

**KARIN SEUFERT**
Untitled

Media: PVC, silver, thread

Photo: Karin Seufert

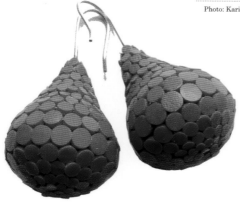

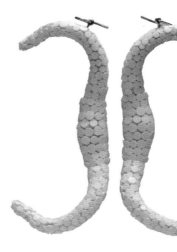

**KARIN SEUFERT**
Untitled

Media: PVC, silver, thread

Photo: Karin Seufert

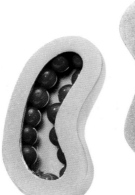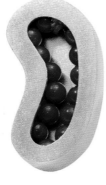

**WALKA STUDIO**
**(Claudia Betancourt & Nano Pulgar)**
Untitled

Media: 950 silver, coral

Photo: Karen Clunes

**LINNÉA ERIKSSON**
Burst

Media: steel, silver

Photo: Linnéa Eriksson

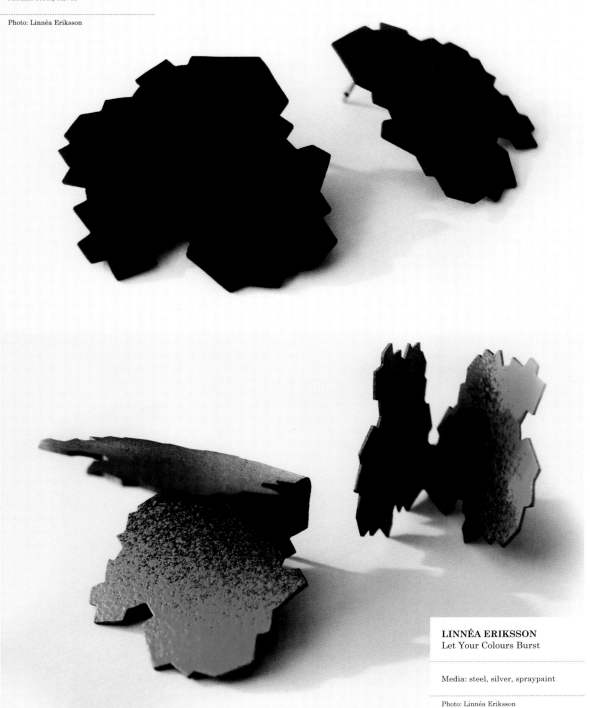

**LINNÉA ERIKSSON**
Let Your Colours Burst

Media: steel, silver, spraypaint

Photo: Linnéa Eriksson

**SARAH WEST**
Infrastructure Series

Media: steel, 925 silver

Photo: Sarah West

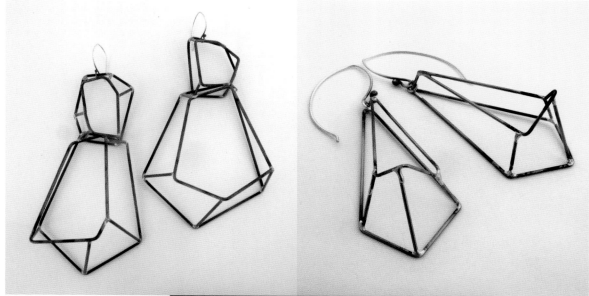

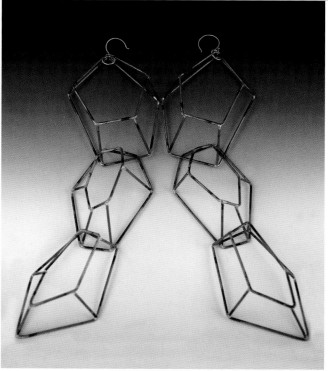

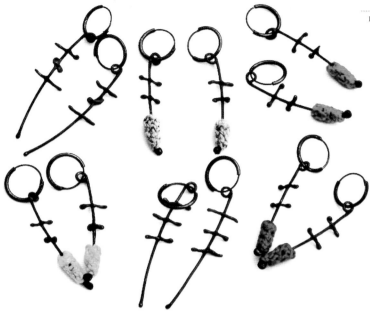

**JOANNE HAYWOOD**
Long Earrings

Media: silver, textile

Photo: Joanne Haywood

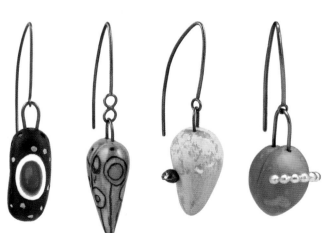

**EMILY WATSON**
Four Earrings

Media: resin clay, 925 silver,
paint, lacquer

Photo: Emily Watson

**ESTER FAIMAN**
Beyond the Era – Rabbits

Media: silver, paint, gold-plated silver

Photo: Katrin Veegen

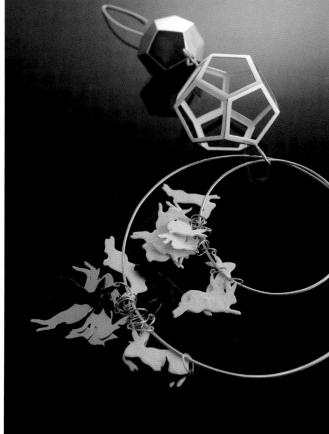

**THERESA BURGER**
Great Grandmother

Media: 925 silver, onyx

Photo: Theresa Burger

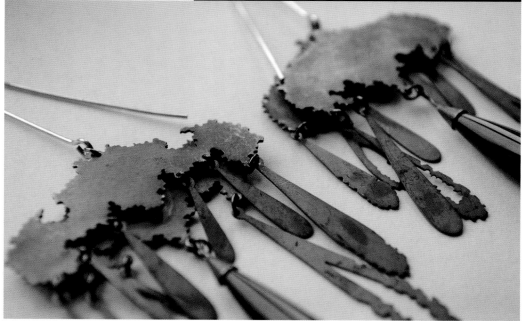

**MEIRI ISHIDA**
Lantern

Media: felt, resin, silver, PMMA

Photo: Meiri Ishida

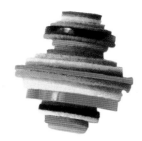

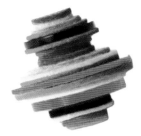

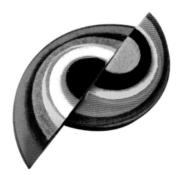

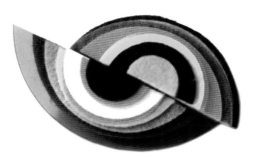

**MEIRI ISHIDA**
Parrot

Media: felt, resin, silver, PMMA

Photo: Meiri Ishida

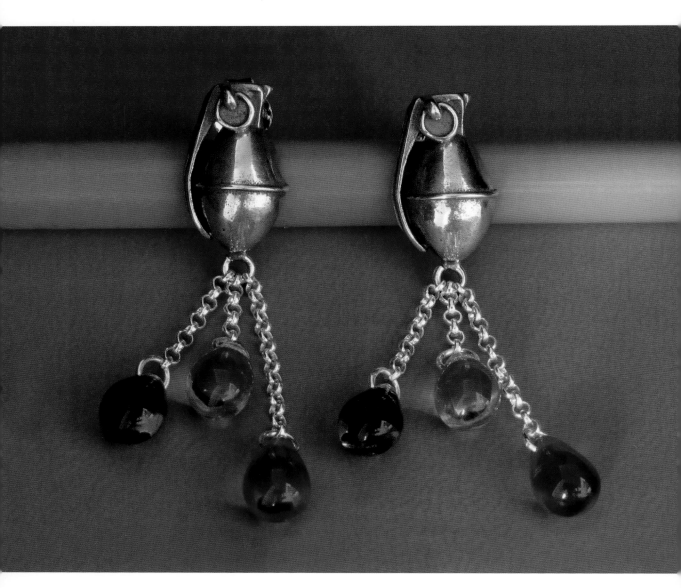

**NICOLAS ESTRADA**
Grenades

Media: silver, crystal

Photo: Nicolas Estrada

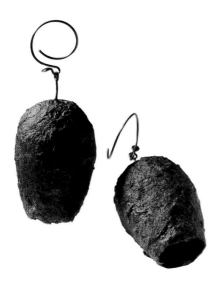

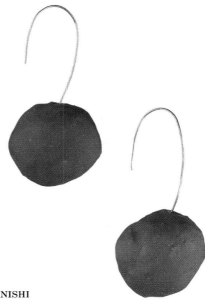

**BIBA SCHUTZ**
Nests

Media: 925 silver, handmade flax
paper, adhesives

Photo: Ron Boszko

**GERALDINE NISHI**
Untitled

Media: concrete, silver

Photo: Federico Cavicchioli

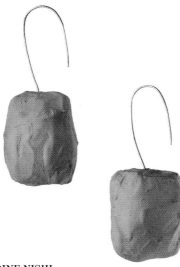

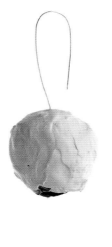

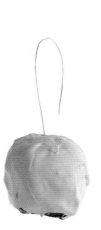

**GERALDINE NISHI**
Untitled

Media: concrete, silver

Photo: Federico Cavicchioli

**GERALDINE NISHI**
Untitled

Media: paper, concrete, silver

Photo: Federico Cavicchioli

**VINA RUST**
Marram Earrings –
Stained Cell Series

Media: 925 silver, 14ct gold

Photo: Doug Yaple

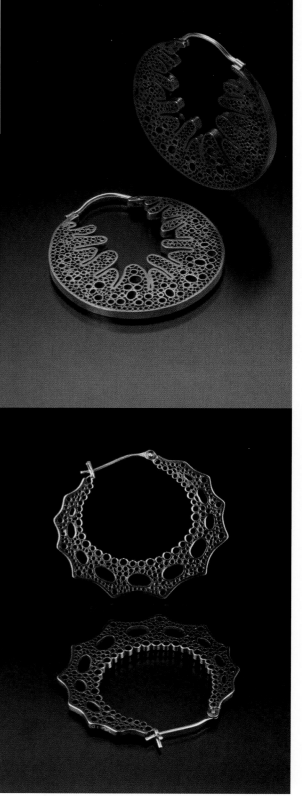

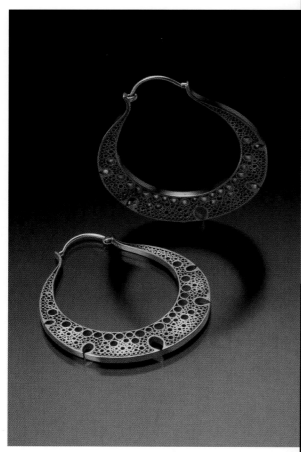

**VINA RUST**
Earrings #10 –
Stained Cell Series

Media: 925 silver, 14ct gold

Photo: Doug Yaple

**VINA RUST**
Earrings #18 –
Stained Cell Series

Media: 925 silver, 14ct gold,
liver of sulphur patina

Photo: Vina Rust

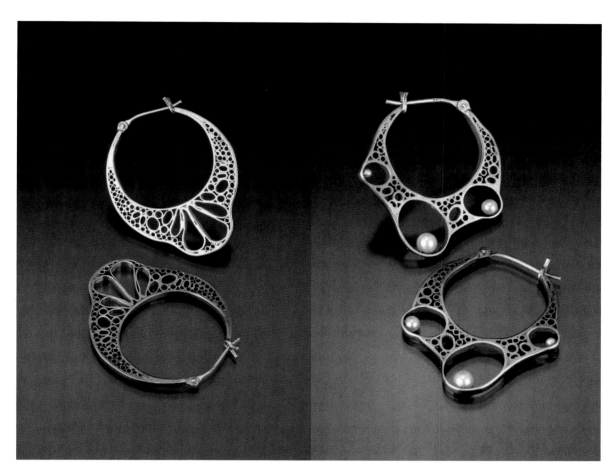

**VINA RUST**
Earrings #15 –
Stained Cell Series

Media: 925 silver, 14ct gold

Photo: Vina Rust

**VINA RUST**
Earrings #1 –
Cysts and Symmetries

Media: 925 silver, 14ct gold,
cultured freshwater pearls

Photo: Vina Rust

**SENAY AKIN**
Faceted Earrings

Media: diamond, 925 silver

Photo: Gokhan Kaya

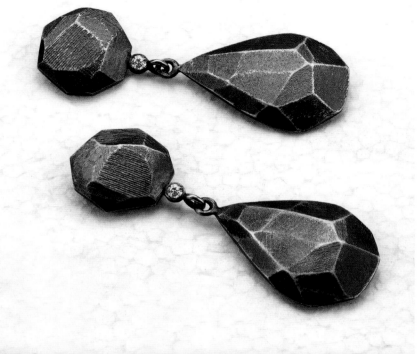

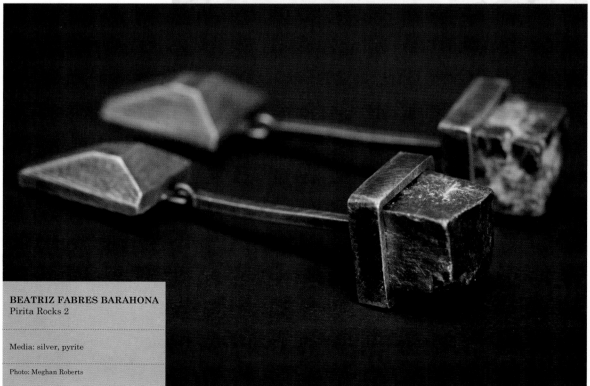

**BEATRIZ FABRES BARAHONA**
Pirita Rocks 2

Media: silver, pyrite

Photo: Meghan Roberts

**VALDIS BROZE**
Smart Earcatcher

Media: 925 silver, 18ct gold, enamel, emerald, pearls, rock crystal

Photo: Maija Muizniece

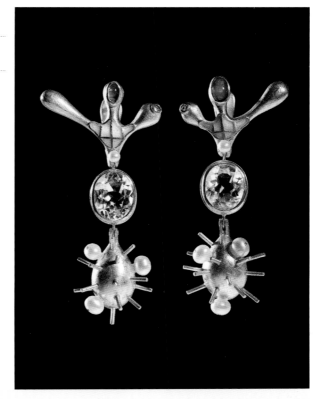

**JACKIE ANDERSON**
Heads Up –
Canadian Mosaic Series

Media: 925 silver, acrylic acetate

Photo: Jackie Anderson

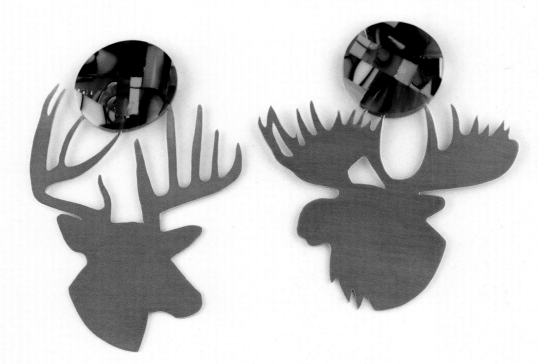

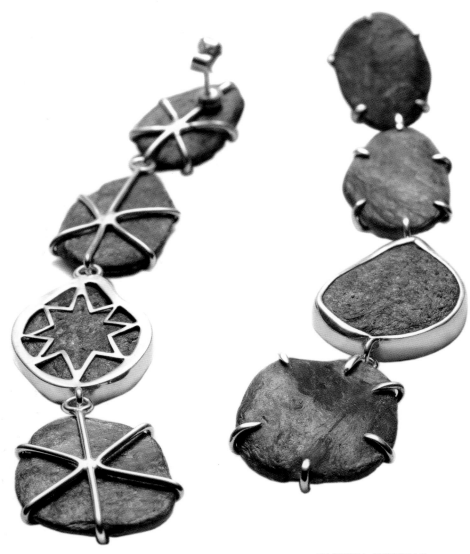

**BARBARA AMZALLAG**
Rock…Star…

Media: 925 silver, fine silver,
freshwater pebbles

Photo: Anthony McLean

**VÍCTOR SALDARRIAGA**
Tr3bejos

Medium: gold

Photo: Andrés Gómez

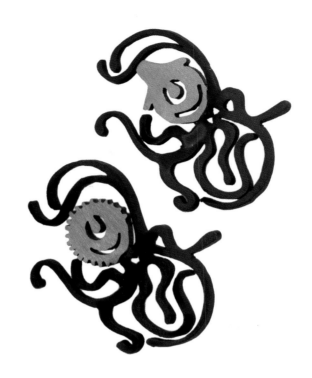

**NATALIA MILOSZ-PIEKARSKA**
Tongue in Cheek

Media: 925 silver, paint

Photo: Natalia Milosz-Piekarska

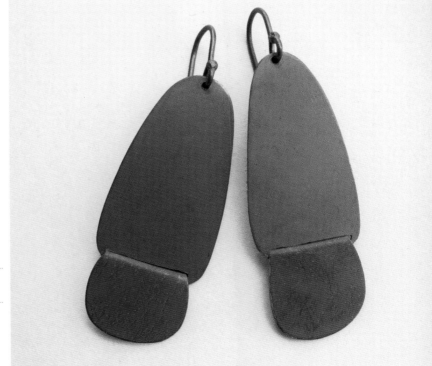

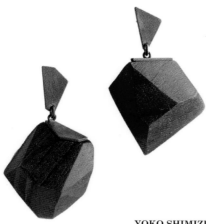

**YOKO SHIMIZU**
Transformation Series – Blue

Media: resin, pigment, silver

Photo: Federico Cavicchioli

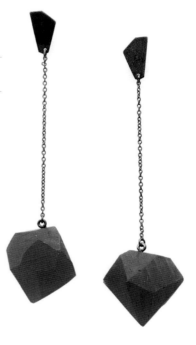

**FANNY AGNIER**
Drops 3

Media: gold, silver, enamel

Photo: Fanny Agnier

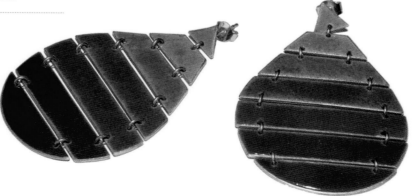

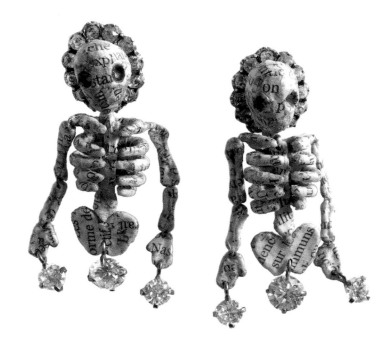

**AURELIE DELLASANTA**
Bling Bling Earrings

Media: papier mâché, metal,
rhinestones, silver

Photo: Aurelie Dellasanta

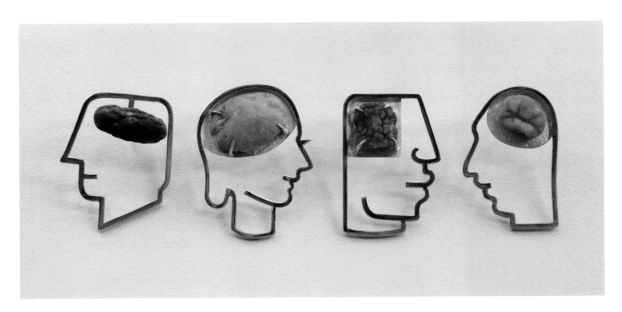

**JUN HU**
Thinking and the Brain

Media: silver, amber

Photo: Jun Hu

**SHARON SCHAFFNER**
Celebration Earrings

Media: 925 silver, onyx, pearls,
red coral, jasper

Photo: Sharon Schaffner

**SHARON SCHAFFNER**
Sputnik Earrings

Medium: 925 silver

Photo: Sharon Schaffner

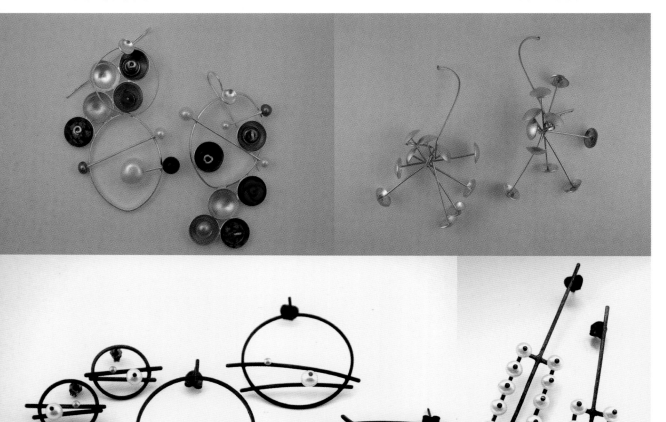

**MARÍA GOTI**
The Old See-Saw

Media: silver, pearls, gold

Photo: María Goti

**MARÍA GOTI**
The Old See-Saw XII

Media: silver, pearls

Photo: María Goti

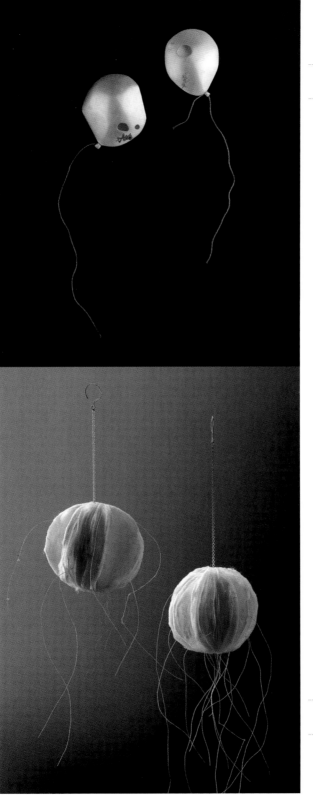

**RUDEE TANCHAROEN**
Untitled

Media: 925 silver, cotton thread

Photo: Federico Cavicchioli

**RUDEE TANCHAROEN**
Dreamer

Media: surgical cotton, silk thread,
18ct gold

Photo: Federico Cavicchioli

**BEATE KLOCKMANN**
Twirls

Media: gold, copper, enamel

Photo: Beate Klockmann

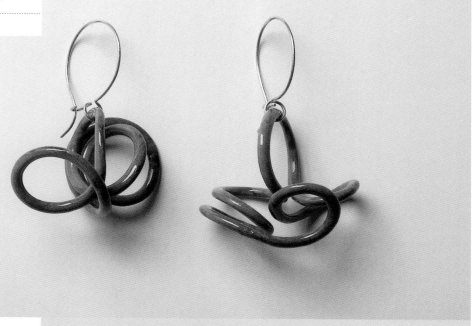

**SUSAN MAY**
Earrings

Medium: 18ct gold

Photo: Susan May

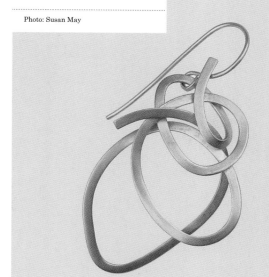
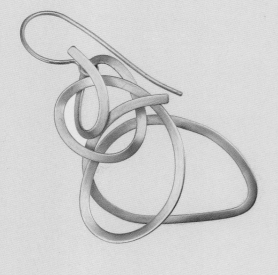

**KARIN SEUFERT**
Untitled

Media: PVC, silver, thread

Photo: Karin Seufert

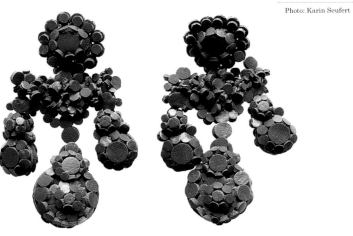

**LAURA EYLES**
From Somewhere You'd Rather Be

Media: 925 silver, cardboard, plastic, sequins

Photo: Andrew Barcham – Screaming Pixel

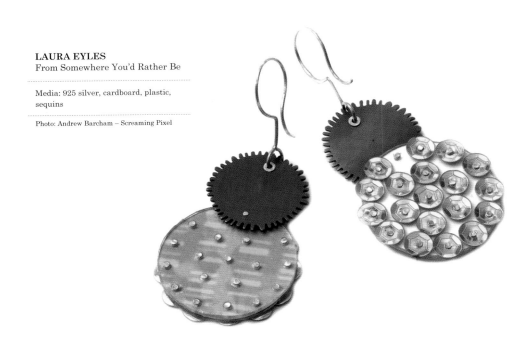

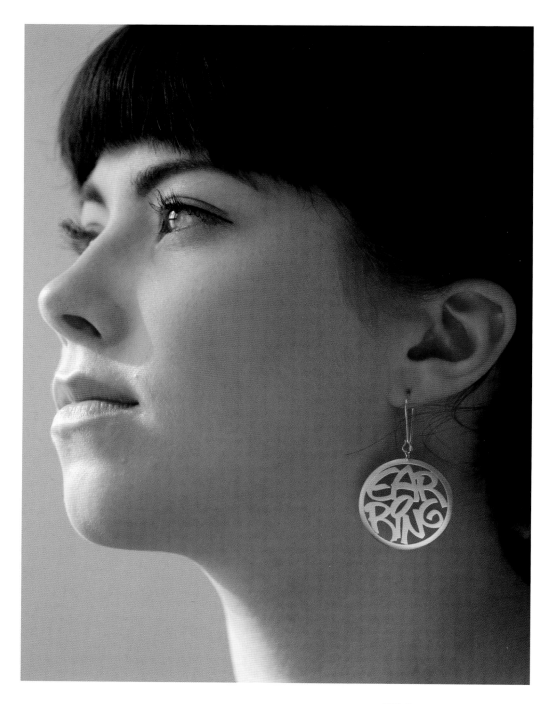

**EERO HINTSANEN**
RingRing – Big Earrings

.............................................................

Medium: 925 silver

.............................................................

Photo: Chao & Eero Jewel

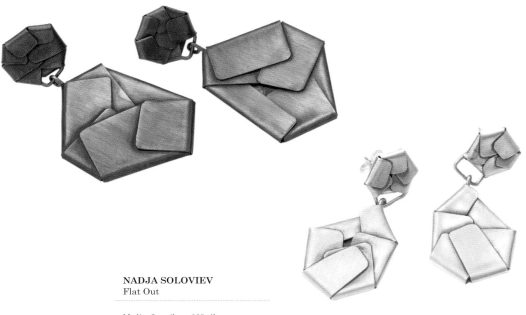

**NADJA SOLOVIEV**
Flat Out

Media: fine silver, 925 silver

Photo: Andrew Barcham & Pieces of
Eight Gallery

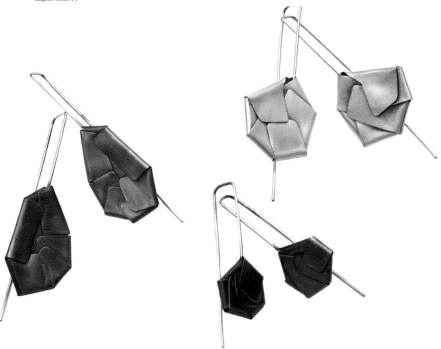

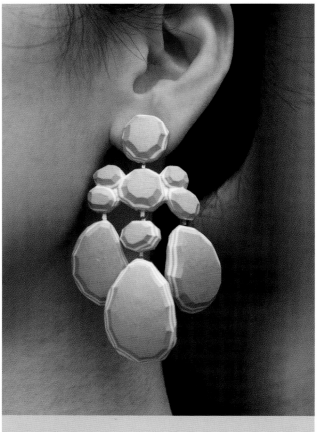

**SHU-LIN WU**
Girandole #2

Media: porcelain, silver

Photo: Hsiao-Yin Chao

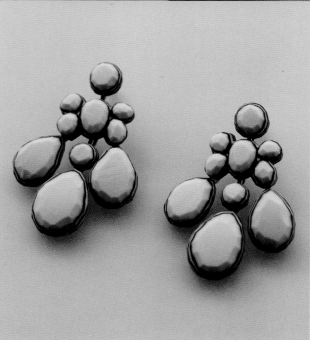

**SHU-LIN WU**
Girandole #9

Media: porcelain, silver

Photo: Shu-Lin Wu

**BIBA SCHUTZ**
Bijoux Cluster

Media: 925 silver, 22ct gold

Photo: Ron Boszko

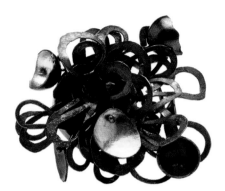
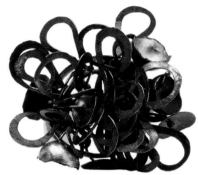

**LARITZA GARCIA**
Viridity

Media: powder-coated copper,
925 silver

Photo: Laritza Garcia

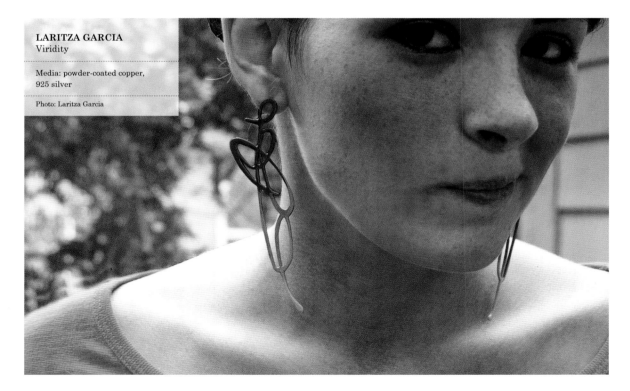

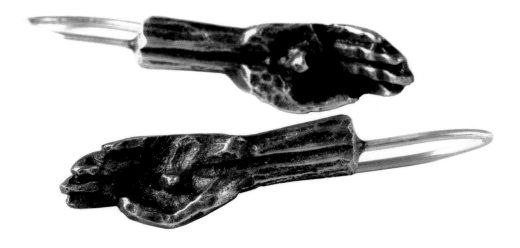

**JORGE MANILLA**
You

Medium: silver

Photo: Bart Vermaercke

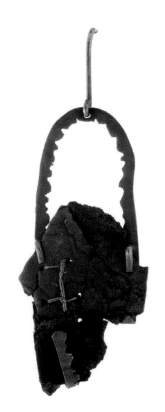

**JORGE MANILLA**
It Was Only A Moment

Media: silver, leather, bioresin, steel

Photo: Donald B. Woodrow

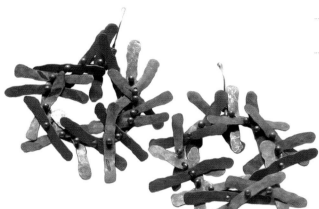

**HUI-MEI PAN**
Chaos

Medium: 925 silver

Photo: Hui-Mei Pan

**BIBA SCHUTZ**
Notes in Motion

Media: 925 silver, 22ct gold

Photo: Ron Boszko

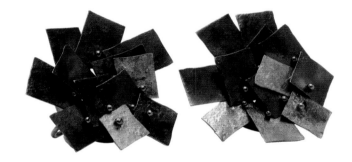

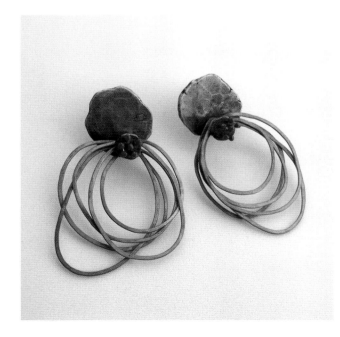

**LIISA HASHIMOTO**
Red Moss Hoop Earring

Media: silver, brass, red enamel paint

Photo: Liisa Hashimoto

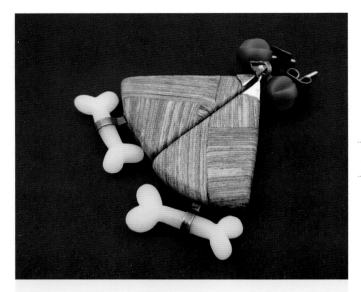

**KVETOSLAVA FLORA
SEKANOVA**
Crossbones

Media: newsprint, PMMA, silver

Photo: Kvetoslava Flora Sekanova

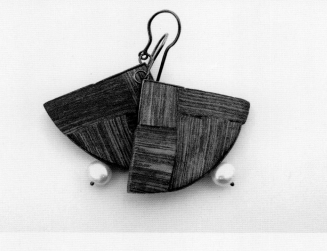

**KVETOSLAVA FLORA
SEKANOVA**
Pearl Earrings

Media: newsprint, silver,
freshwater pearls

Photo: Kvetoslava Flora Sekanova

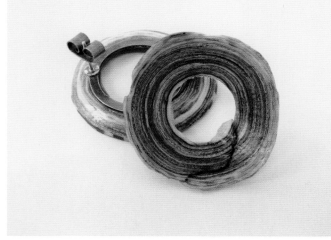

**KVETOSLAVA FLORA
SEKANOVA**
Circle

Media: newsprint, silver

Photo: Kvetoslava Flora Sekanova

**ENRIC MAJORAL**
Exclusive Piece

Media: white gold, acrylic paint

Photo: Majoral

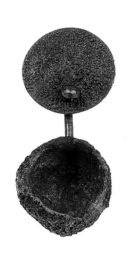
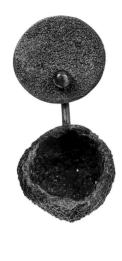

**ANDREA CODERCH VALOR**
Hana 2

Media: silver, shibuichi

Photo: Andrea Coderch Valor

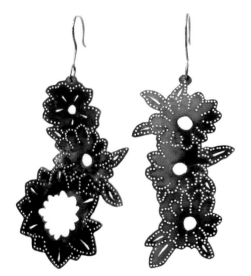

**ANDREA CODERCH VALOR**
Hana

Media: gold, silver, shibuichi,
kimono silk

Photo: Andrea Coderch Valor

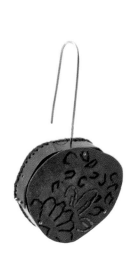
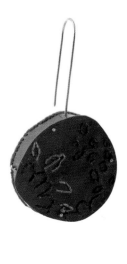

## ÅSA ELMSTAM
Tags

Medium: silver

Photo: Åsa Elmstam

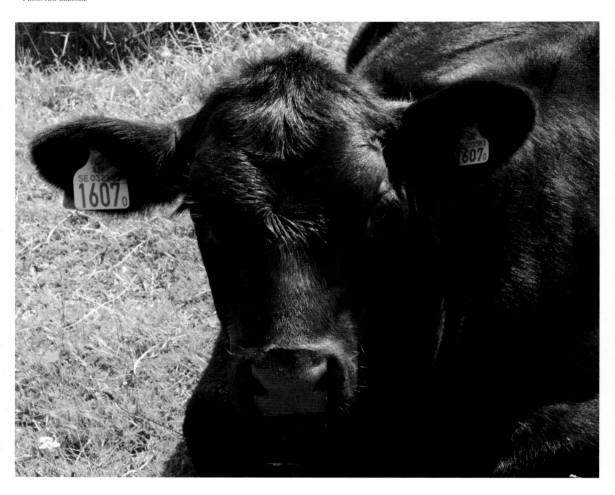

## LIESBET BUSSCHE
Urban Jewelry

Medium: brass

Photo: Liesbet Bussche

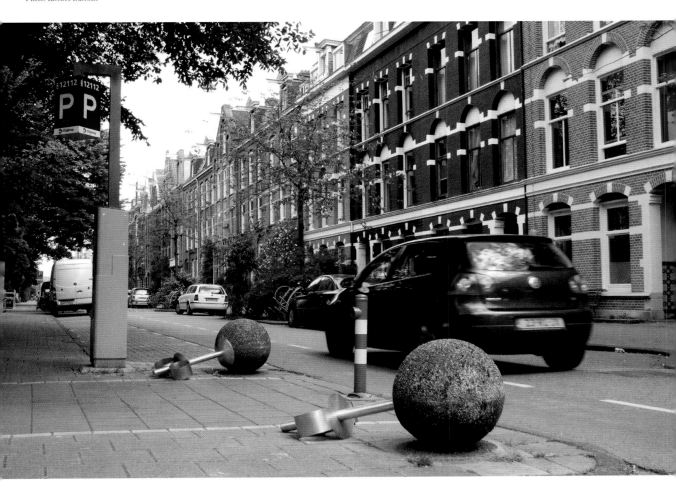

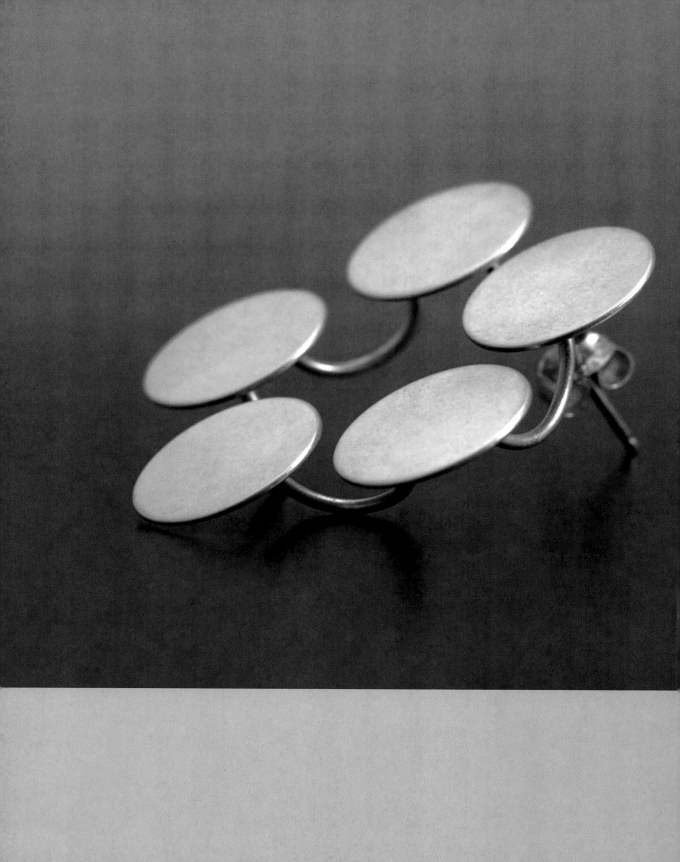

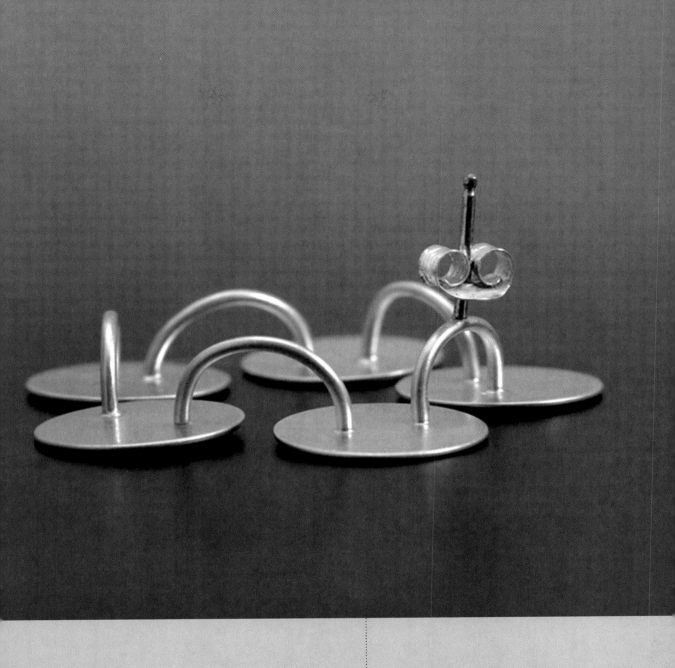

DELICATE

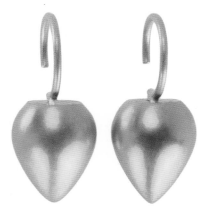

**CHRISTA LÜHTJE**
Untitled

Medium: gold

Photo: Eva Jünger

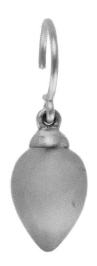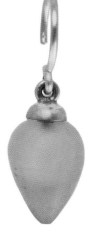

**CHRISTA LÜHTJE**
Untitled

Media: gold, aquamarine

Photo: Eva Jünger

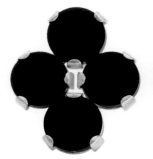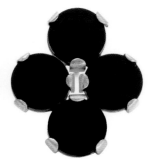

**CHRISTA LÜHTJE**
Untitled

Media: gold, onyx

Photo: Eva Jünger

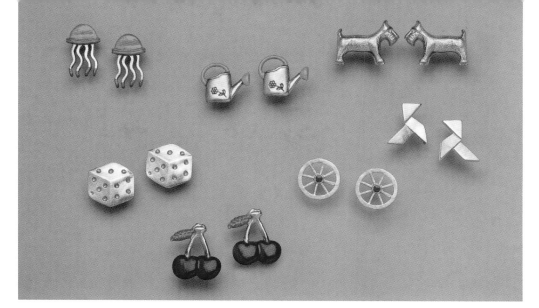

**XAVIER MONCLÚS**
Dinky Jewels

Media: silver, enamel paint

Photo: Xavier Monclús

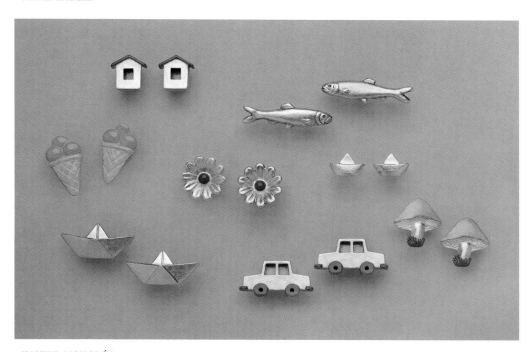

**XAVIER MONCLÚS**
Dinky Jewels

Media: silver, enamel paint

Photo: Xavier Monclús

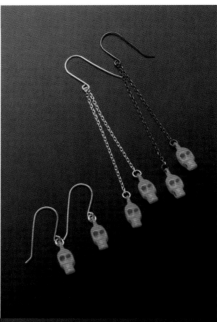

**TINA LILIENTHAL**
Fluoro Skull Earrings

Media: silver, powder-coated silver

Photo: Joel Degen

**TINA LILIENTHAL**
Strawberry & Skull Earrings

Media: polyester resin, silver

Photo: Joel Degen

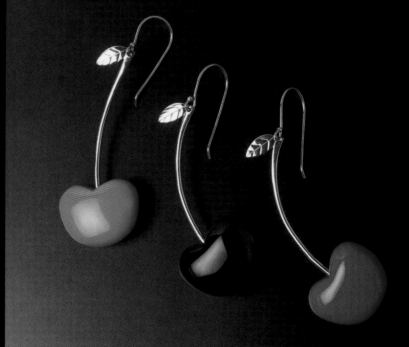

**TINA LILIENTHAL**
Cherry Earrings

Media: polyester resin, silver

Photo: Joel Degen

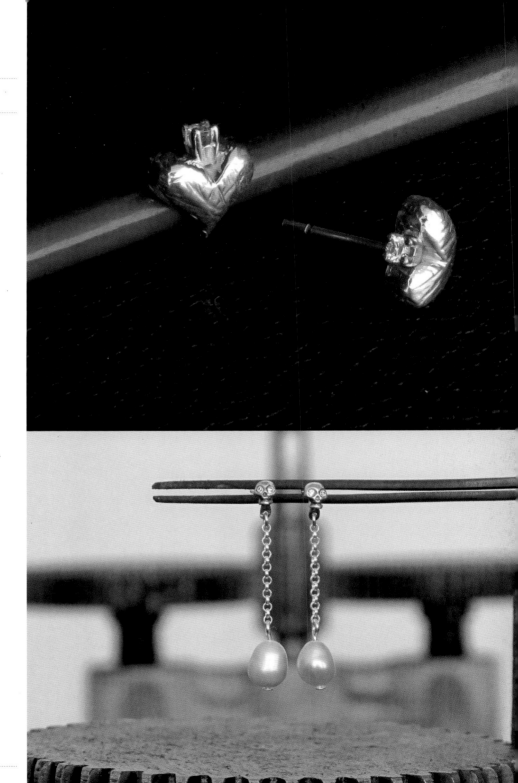

**NICOLAS ESTRADA**
Hearts

Media: gold, diamonds

Photo: Nicolas Estrada

**NICOLAS ESTRADA**
Skulls

Media: silver, crystal, pearls

Photo: Nicolas Estrada

**JOANNE HAYWOOD**
Juniper Studs

Medium: silver

Photo: Joanne Haywood

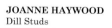

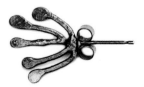

**JOANNE HAYWOOD**
Dill Studs

Medium: silver

Photo: Joanne Haywood

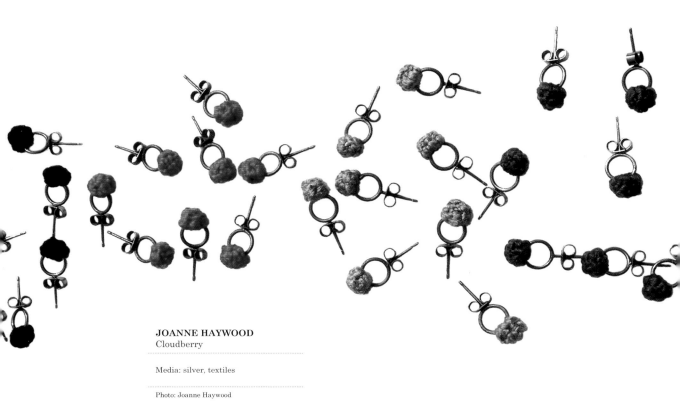

**JOANNE HAYWOOD**
Cloudberry

Media: silver, textiles

Photo: Joanne Haywood

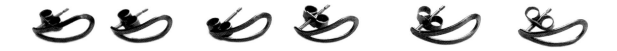

**JOANNE HAYWOOD**
Omega Studs

Medium: silver

Photo: Joanne Haywood

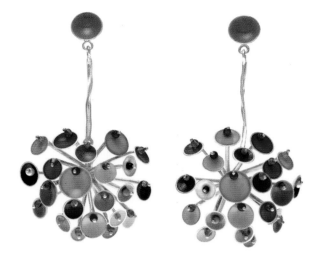

**ADRIANA HENAO MEJÍA**
Emergence – Vaivén

Media: 950 silver, glazed enamel,
turquoise, lapis lazuli, garnet,
cornelian, onyx, pearl

Photo: Jorge Mario Múnera

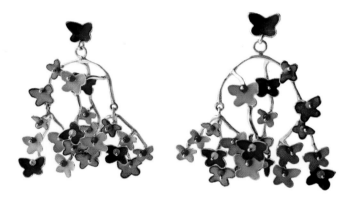

**ADRIANA HENAO MEJÍA**
Migrations – Vaivén

Media: 950 silver, glazed enamel,
cornelian, rose quartz, turquoise

Photo: Jorge Mario Múnera

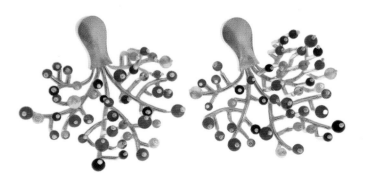

**ADRIANA HENAO MEJÍA**
Tree of Life – Arbórea

Media: 950 silver, cornelian, garnet,
turquoise, onyx, amethyst, pearls
jadeite, amber

Photo: Jorge Mario Múnera

**ANDREA VELÁZQUEZ
CALLEJA**
Keum-boo 9

Media: 925 silver, 24ct gold,
lapis lazuli, keum-boo

Photo: Andrea Velázquez Calleja

**ANDREA VELÁZQUEZ
CALLEJA**
Keum-boo 5

Media: 925 silver, 24ct gold,
magnetite, keum-boo

Photo: Andrea Velázquez Calleja

**ANDREA VELÁZQUEZ
CALLEJA**
Keum-boo 10

Media: 925 silver, 24ct gold,
magnetite, keum-boo

Photo: Andrea Velázquez Calleja

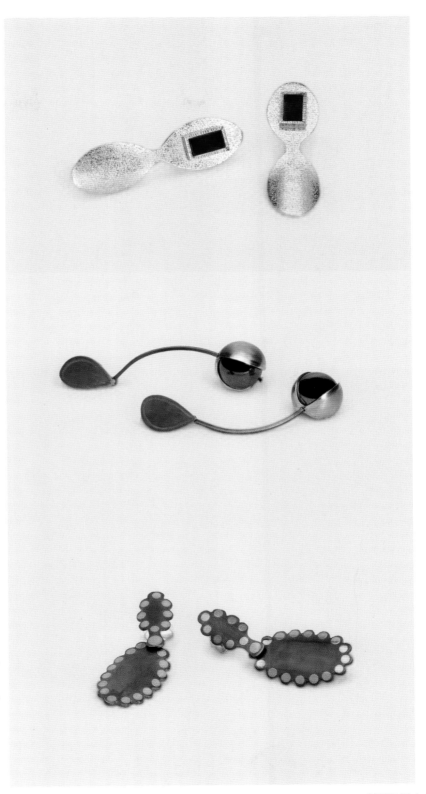

**MARINA BABIĆ**
Long Stem Rose Earrings

Media: 925 silver, acrylic paint

Photo: Digital by Design – Paul Ambtman

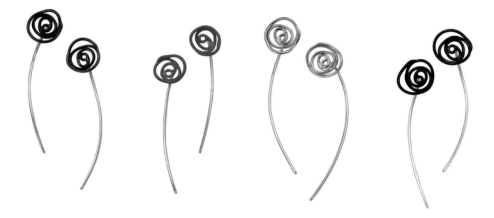

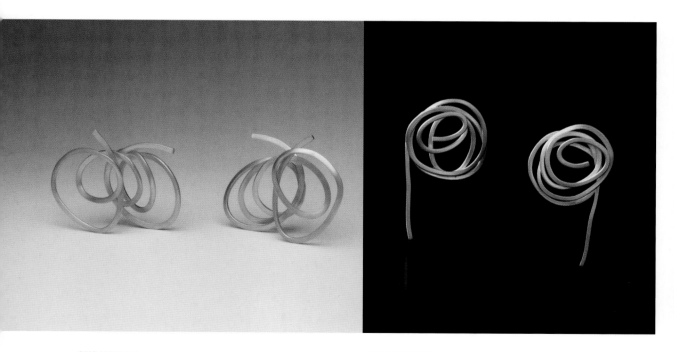

**SUSAN MAY**
Pouch Earrings

Medium: 925 silver

Photo: Joël Degen

**SUSAN MAY**
Earrings

Medium: 18ct gold

Photo: Goldsmiths' Company London

## PILAR COTTER
Petit Lies

Media: porcelain, gold

Photo: Pilar Cotter

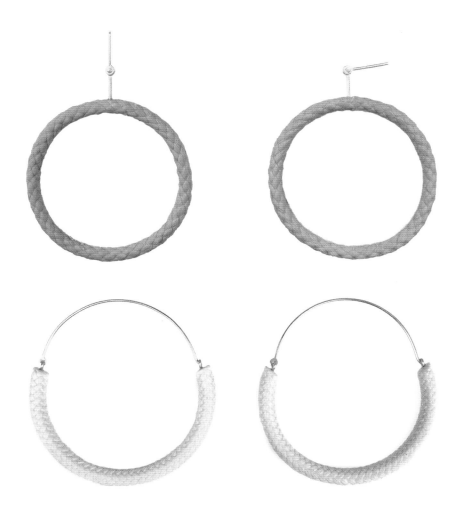

**MARTA SÀNCHEZ OMS**
Fusinos Conus

Media: silver, natural conus shell

Photo: Marta Sànchez Oms

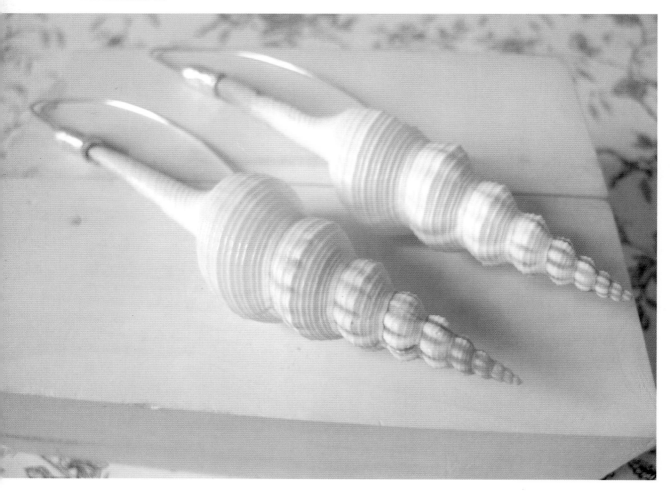

**SAMUEL SAAVEDRA**
Carousel

Media: 18ct gold, cultured
pearls

Photo: Montse Poch

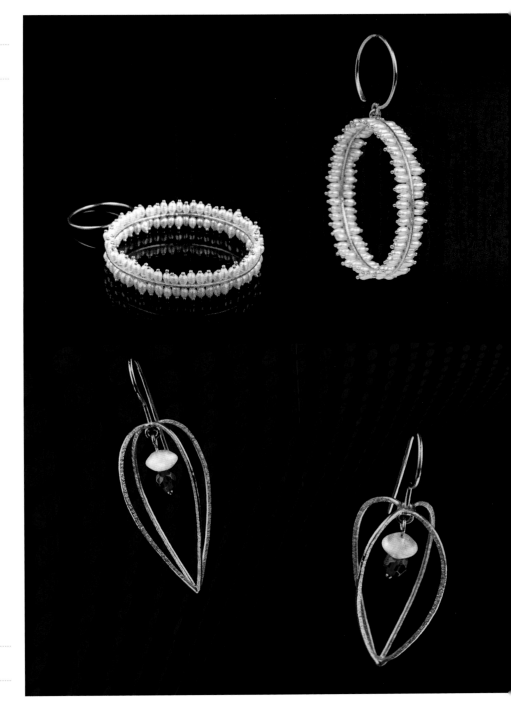

**SAMUEL SAAVEDRA**
Tulip

Media: 18ct gold, garnet,
rose quartz

Photo: Montse Poch

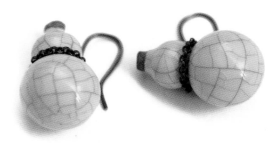

**PETER HOOGEBOOM**
Jugs Ear Jewels

Media: ceramics, silver, cork

Photo: Peter Hoogeboom

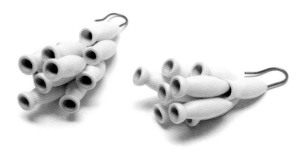

**PETER HOOGEBOOM**
North Sea Ear Jewels White

Media: fused ceramics, silver

Photo: Francis Willemstijn

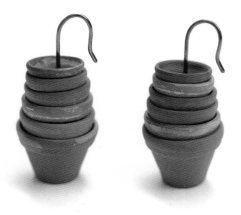

**PETER HOOGEBOOM**
Flowerpots Ear Jewels

Media: terracotta, silver

Photo: Peter Hoogeboom

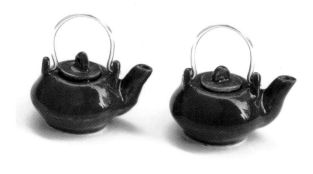

**PETER HOOGEBOOM**
Teapots Ear Jewels Green

Media: porcelain, silver

Photo: Peter Hoogeboom

**TERRY WARE**
Bespoke Carved Coral Earrings

.................................................

Media: antique Italian hand-carved
Mediterranean coral, 18ct yellow gold,
white diamonds

.................................................

Photo: Carin Krasner.com

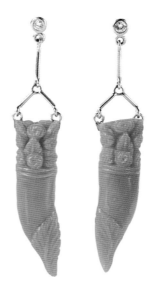

**TERRY WARE**
Bespoke Duke di Urbino Earrings

.................................................

Media: antique Italian hand-carved
Mediterranean coral, 18ct rose gold,
diamond quatrefoil

.................................................

Photo: Carin Krasner.com

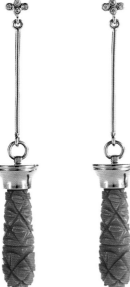
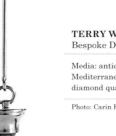

**TERRY WARE**
Single Fly Earrings

.................................................

Media: Persian turquoise drops,
diamonds, 18ct rose gold

.................................................

Photo: Carin Krasner.com

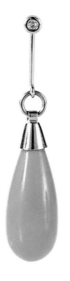
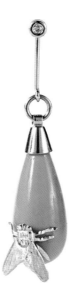

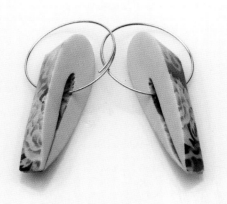

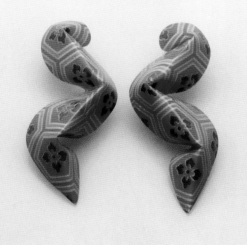

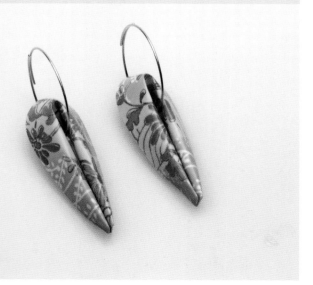

**MARLENE BEYER**
Origami

Media: handmade plastics, hand
printed with Japanese patterns

Photo: Marlene Beyer

**WALKA STUDIO**
**(Claudia Betancourt & Nano Pulgar)**
Horsehair Shoots

Media: 950 silver, horsehair, vegetable fibre

Photo: Karen Clunes

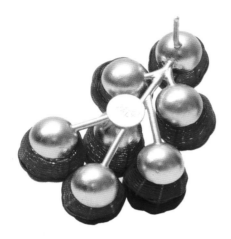
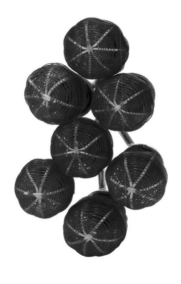

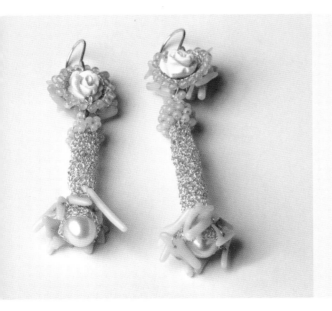
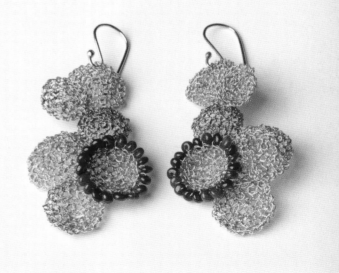

**SU KROKER**
Little Pies

Media: 18ct gold, raw diamonds,
Tahitian pearls

Photo: Frans Bouwmeester Fotografie

**SU KROKER**
Fleur d'Or

Media: 24ct gold, 18ct gold,
18ct white gold, ruby

Photo: Frans Bouwmeester Fotografie

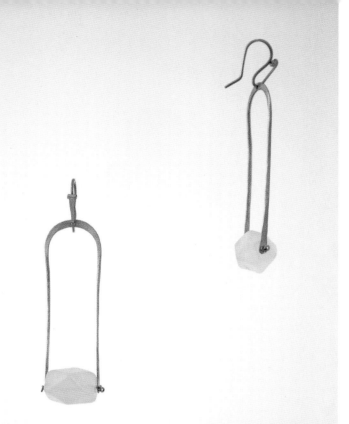

**CUCÚ RUIZ**
Arc

Media: gold, agate

Photo: Cucú Ruiz

**IRO KASKANI**
The Space in Between

Medium: 925 silver

Photo: Dimitris Vattis

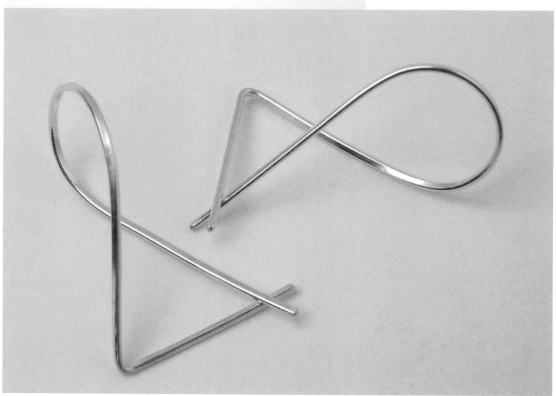

**DENISE QUEIROZ**
Bird

Medium: 950 silver

Photo: Marcos Vianna

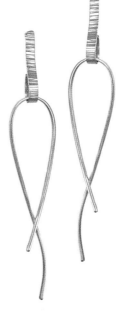

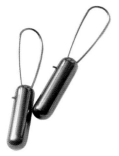

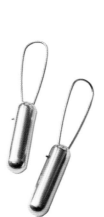

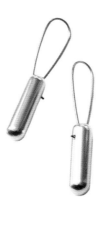

**LAURA EYLES**
Capsule Earrings

Media: 925 silver, stainless steel,
gold-plated

Photo: Andrew Barcham – Screaming Pixel

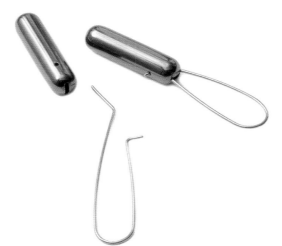

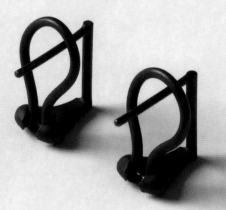

**MARC MONZÓ**
Omega

Medium: silver

Photo: Marc Monzó

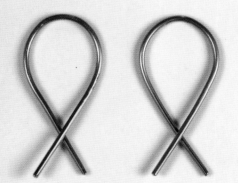

**MARC MONZÓ**
X Earrings

Medium: 18ct gold

Photo: Marc Monzó

**MARC MONZÓ**
Fire

Medium: 18ct gold

Photo: Marc Monzó

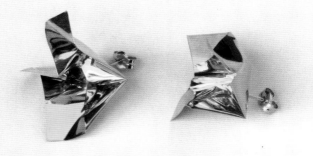

**MARC MONZÓ**
1 mm

Medium: 18ct gold

Photo: Marc Monzó

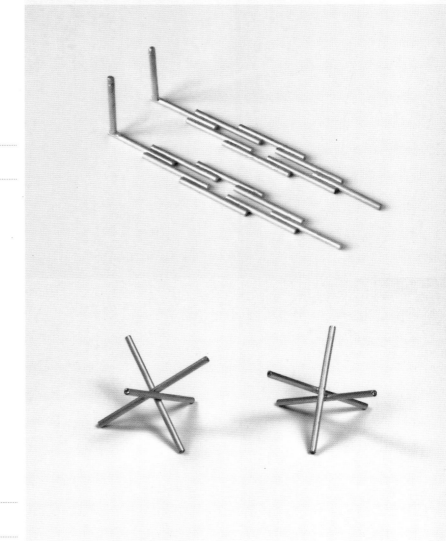

**MARC MONZÓ**
Star

Media: 18ct gold, diamonds

Photo: Marc Monzó

**JÚLIA COMPTE**
Cactus

Medium: silver

Photo: Elisenda Compte

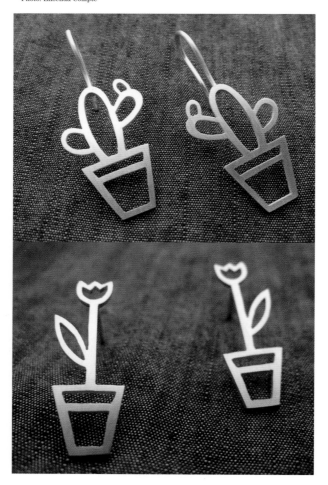

**JÚLIA COMPTE**
Flower

Medium: silver

Photo: Elisenda Compte

**ANGELA BUBASH**
Fin #4

Media: 925 silver, glass,
dyed feathers

Photo: Jonathan Heller

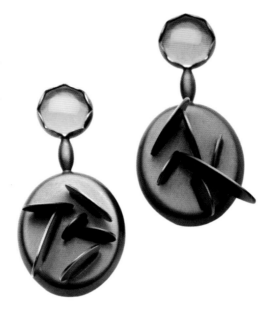

**CONSTANZA SOTO DONOSO**
Pruning

Media: 940 silver, red cotton thread

Photo: Constanza Soto Donoso

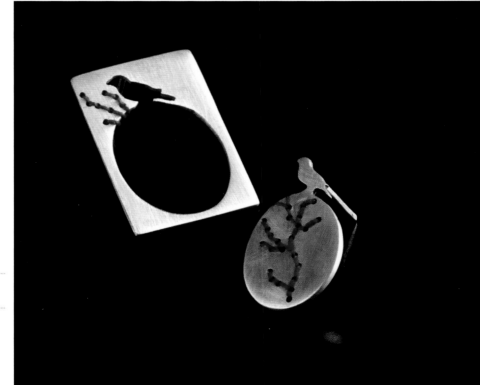

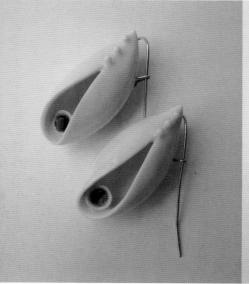

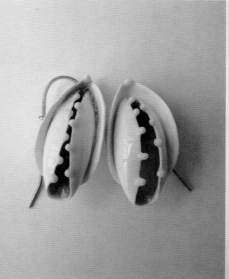

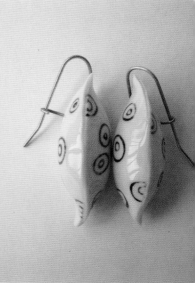

**ANNE PERBET JACKSON**
Droplet

Media: porcelain, coloured glass, silver

Photo: Anne Perbet Jackson

**ANNE PERBET JACKSON**
Oyster

Media: porcelain, coloured glass, silver

Photo: Anne Perbet Jackson

**ANNE PERBET JACKSON**
Mussel

Media: porcelain, copper oxide, silver

Photo: Anne Perbet Jackson

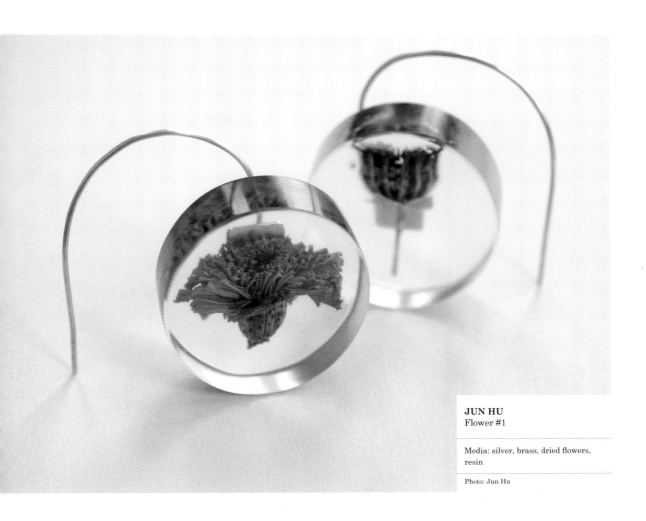

**JUN HU**
Flower #1

Media: silver, brass, dried flowers, resin

Photo: Jun Hu

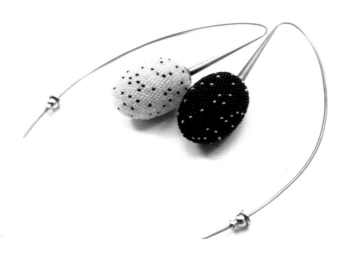

**JACQUELINE I. LILLIE**
Swivel Earrings

Media: titanium, glass beads

Photo: Petr Dvorak

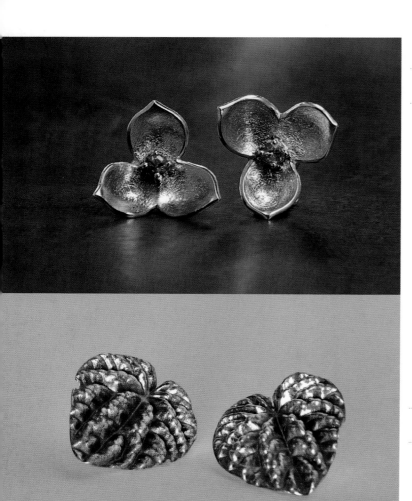

**SANDRA PONTNOU FERRER**
Seed

Media: 925 silver, 18ct gold,
aquamarine

Photo: Eva Diez

**MANUELA URIBE**
Oxidized Leaves

Medium: 925 silver

Photo: Luciano Uribe

**MISUN WON**
Coral Flower Earrings

Media: 925 silver, coral, pearl

Photo: Misun Won

**SAYUMI YOKOUCHI**
Two Structures

Media: silver, found wire, minerals, thread

Photo: Elizabeth Waugh

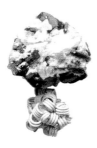
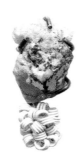
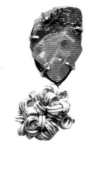
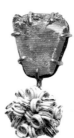

**SAYUMI YOKOUCHI**
Two Structures

Media: silver, found wire, minerals, thread

Photo: Elizabeth Waugh

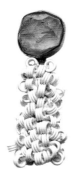
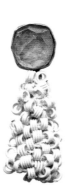
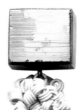

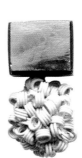

## LEONOR HIPÓLITO
Splendour of Wearability

Medium: silver

Photo: Arne Kaiser

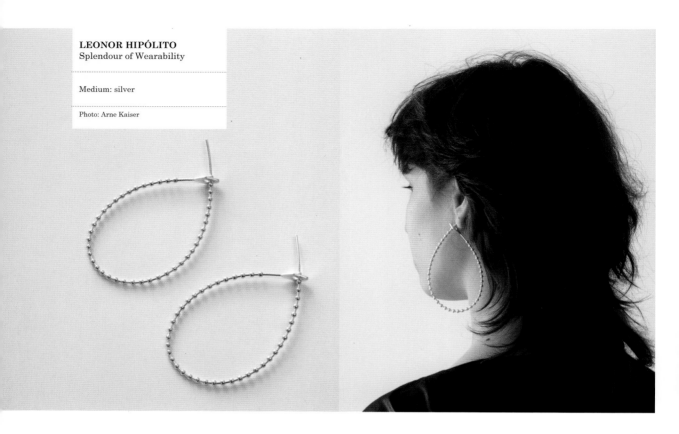

## LEONOR HIPÓLITO
Heritage

Media: silver, picture

Photo: Arne Kaiser

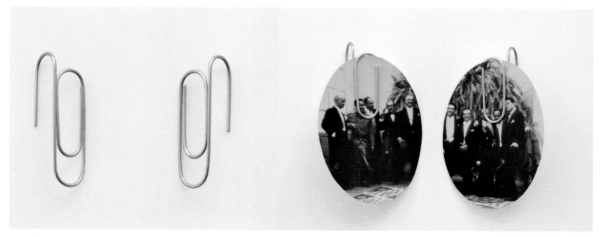

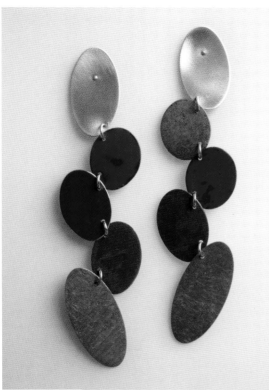

**ESTELA GUITART**
Lightweight

Media: silver, Japanese urushi
lacquer, gold leaf

Photo: Estela Guitart

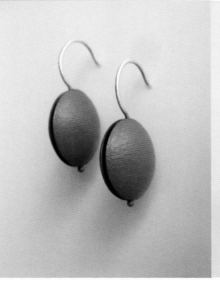

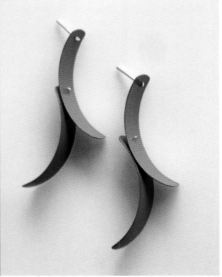

**ESTELA GUITART**
N9

Media: silver, Japanese urushi
lacquer

Photo: Estela Guitart

**ESTELA GUITART**
Module

Media: silver, Japanese urushi
lacquer

Photo: Estela Guitart

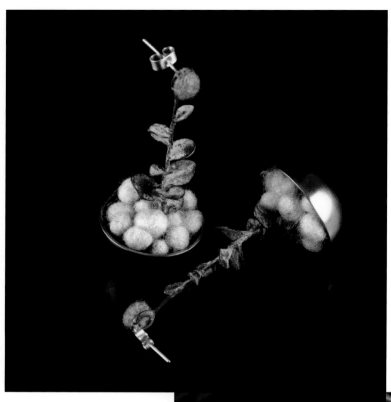

**CONSTANZA SOTO DONOSO**
Good Seed

Media: 940 silver, copper, sheep's wool

Photo: Constanza Soto Donoso

**GABRIELA BARRÓN OLVERA**
Fishing in the River Nazas

Medium: silver

Photo: Carlos Maqueda

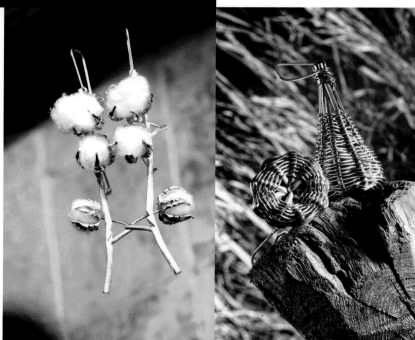

**GABRIELA BARRÓN OLVERA**
White Gold of the Desert

Media: silver, cotton

Photo: Carlos Maqueda

**GILLIAN E. BATCHER**
Fold Over Sprockets

Media: stainless steel, 925 silver,
pearls

Photo: Paul Ambtman

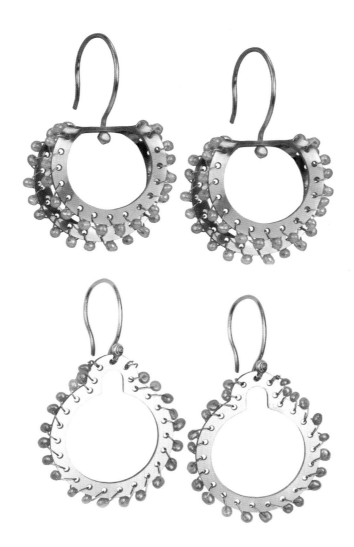

**GILLIAN E. BATCHER**
Sprocket Drops

Media: stainless steel, 18ct yellow
gold, pearls

Photo: Paul Ambtman

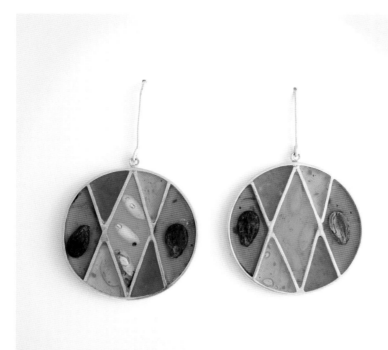

**JULIANA ESTRADA LONDOÑO**
Little Fruits

Media: 975 silver, resins, fruit seeds,
semi-precious stones

Photo: Juliana Estrada Londoño

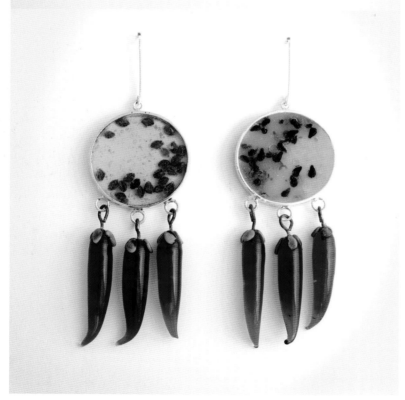

**JULIANA ESTRADA LONDOÑO**
Deseeded Chillis

Media: 975 silver, resins, fruit seeds,
semi-precious stones

Photo: Juliana Estrada Londoño

## ENRIC MAJORAL
Neptune Grass

Media: silver, gold

Photo: Majoral

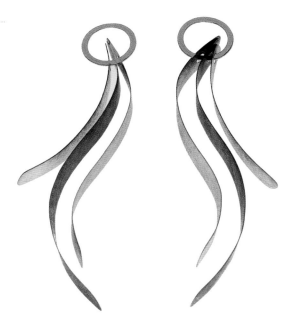

## BLANCA SÁNCHEZ
Untitled – Brilliant

Medium: silver

Photo: Blanca Sánchez

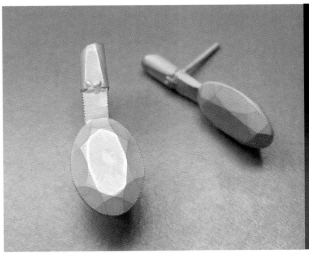

## ALINE KOKINOPOULOS
Lilac

Media: silver, synthetic enamel

Photo: Aline Kokinopoulos

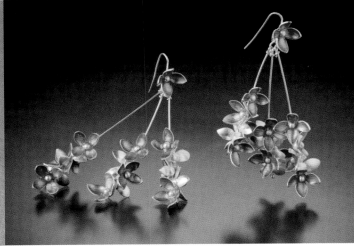

**MARÍA LILIANA RUIZ**
Do You Fancy Some Tea?

Medium: 925 silver

Photo: Lirú

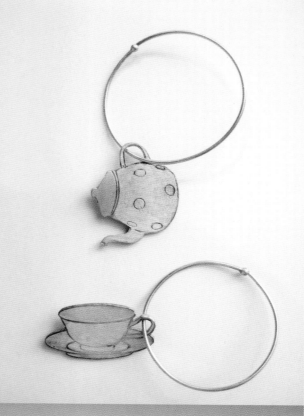

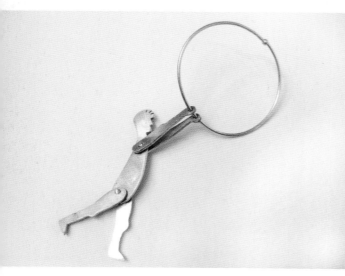

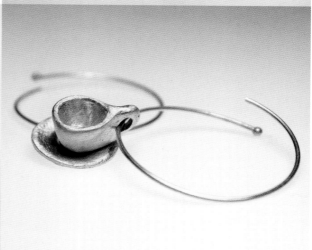

**MARÍA LILIANA RUIZ**
Little Man

Medium: 925 silver

Photo: Lirú

**MARÍA LILIANA RUIZ**
He, She

Medium: 925 silver

Photo: Lirú

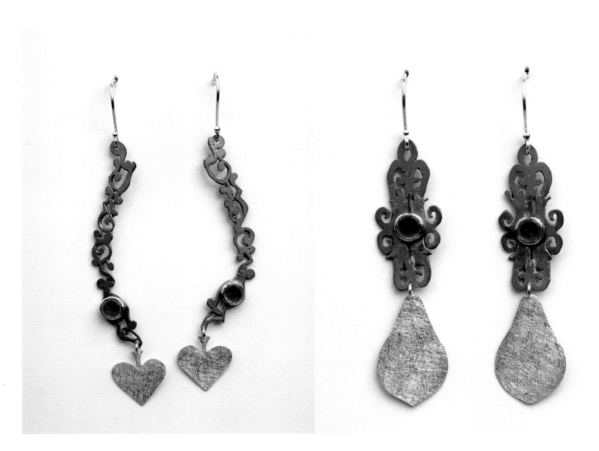

**CARLES SERRANO – DELAJOIA**
Antea XVI

Media: silver, 18ct green gold, rubellite

Photo: Carles Serrano

**CARLES SERRANO – DELAJOIA**
Antea XXXII

Media: silver, 18ct green gold, rubellite

Photo: Carles Serrano

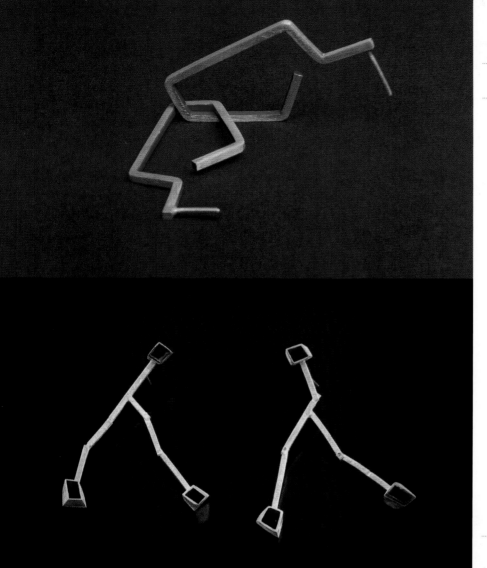

**MAGALÍ ANIDJAR**
Geometrics

Media: 925 silver, cold enamel

Photo: Cecilia Kelly

**MARÍA DEL MAR SÁNCHEZ**
Walkers I

Media: silver, acrylic paint

Photo: Creativalente

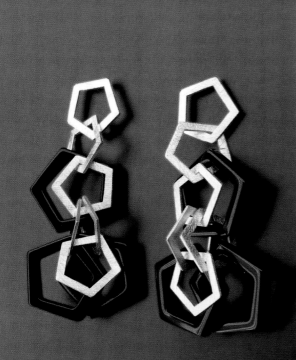

**BABETTE VON DOHNANYI**
Movement

Media: 925 silver, onyx

Photo: Federico Cavicchioli

**LIAUNG-CHUNG YEN**
Stone #3

Media: 18ct gold, pearls

Photo: Liaung-Chung Yen

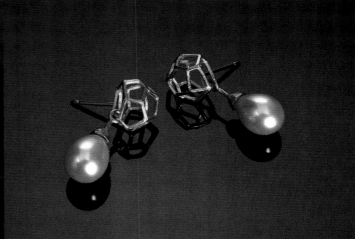

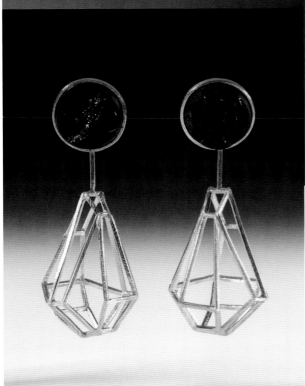

**LIAUNG-CHUNG YEN**
Stone #2

Media: 18ct gold, black
tourmalines

Photo: Liaung-Chung Yen

**BEATE KLOCKMANN**
Untitled

Media: gold, enamel

Photo: Beate Klockmann

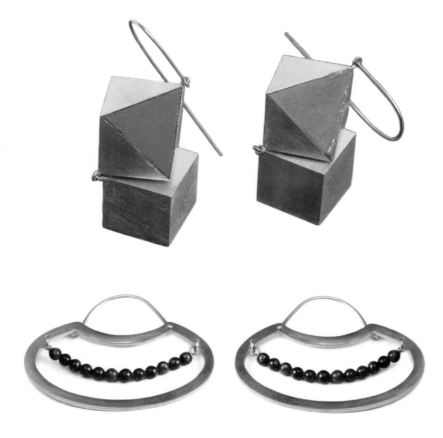

**WALKA STUDIO**
**(Claudia Betancourt & Nano Pulgar)**
Souvenir

Media: gold-plated 950 silver, lapis lazuli

Photo: Karen Clunes

**CARACTÈRE**
**(Gema Barrera & Pascal Cretin)**
Diabolo

Media: silver, PVC suction cups,
medical steel

Photo: Caractère

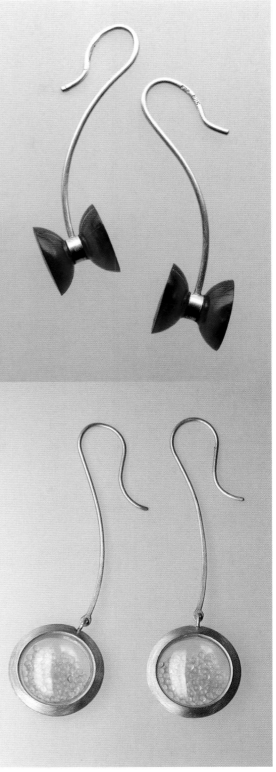

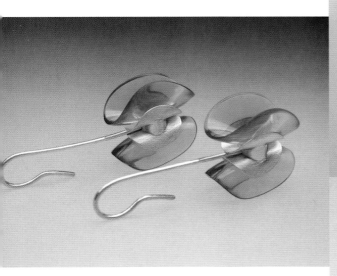

**CARACTÈRE**
**(Gema Barrera & Pascal Cretin)**
Butterflies

Media: silver, PVC suction cups,
medical steel

Photo: Caractère

**CARACTÈRE**
**(Gema Barrera & Pascal Cretin)**
DoReMiFaSol

Media: silver, glass, glass beads

Photo: Caractère

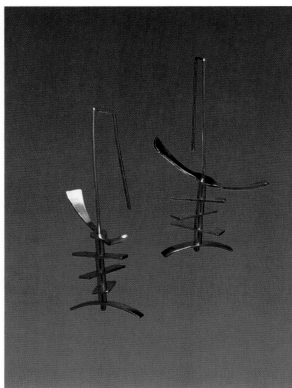

**JOSEP RAVENTÓS**
Japan House

Medium: 925 silver

Photo: Josep Raventós

**SELMA LEAL**
Life Collection

Media: gold, silver, enamel

Photo: Gilmar Nashiro

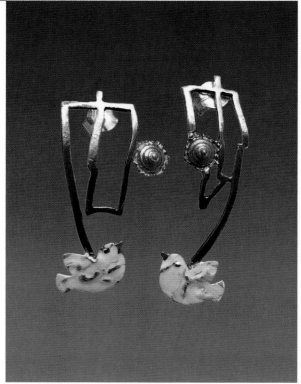

**CARMEN PINTOR – GALERÍA
MEKO JOYERÍA DE AUTOR**
Memories of Barcelona

Media: sea glass, 18ct gold, diamonds

Photo: Carmen Pintor

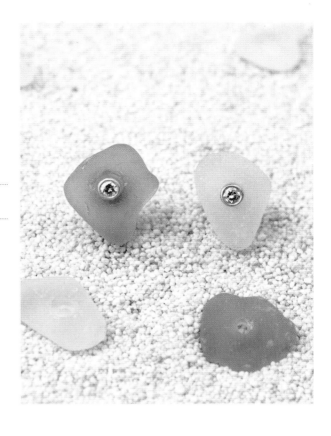

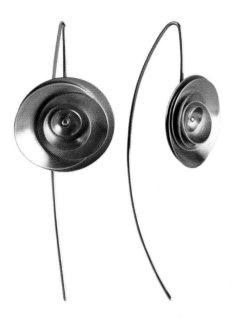

**ANNE BADER**
Orbit

Medium: 925 silver

Photo: Stefano Zanini

**MARÍA SOLÓRZANO**
Biblis

Media: 925 silver, leather, Tyvek®

Photo: Maria Solórzano

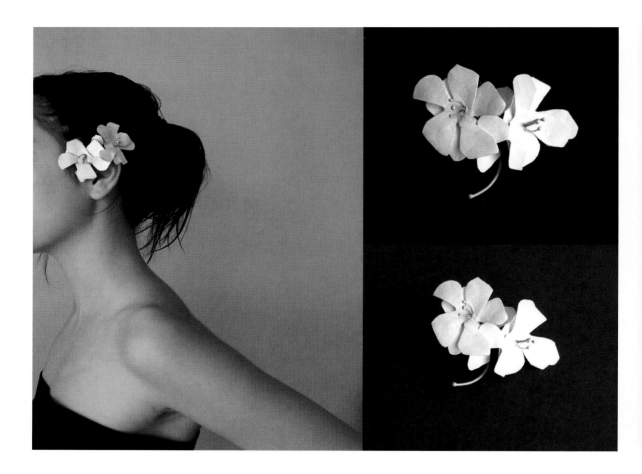

**JUDY McCAIG**
Two Birds and Black Tree

Media: silver, PMMA, paint,
gold leaf

Photo: Richard Matzinger

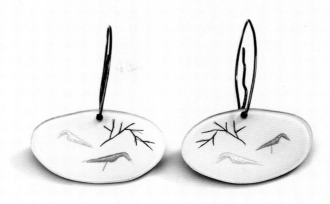

**JUDY McCAIG**
Black Birds

Media: silver, Formica, paint

Photo: Richard Matzinger

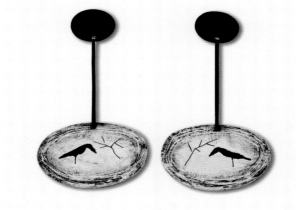

**JUDY McCAIG**
Golden Bird

Media: silver, PMMA, paint,
gold leaf

Photo: Richard Matzinger

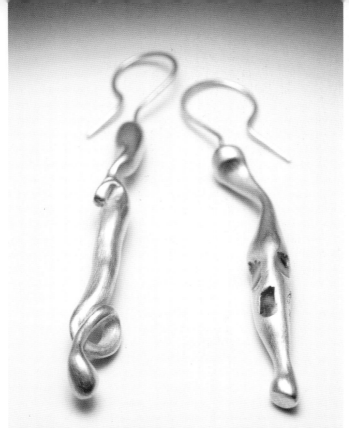

**FRANCE ROY**
Mankind

Media: 925 silver, coloured
epoxy resin

Photo: Anthony McLean

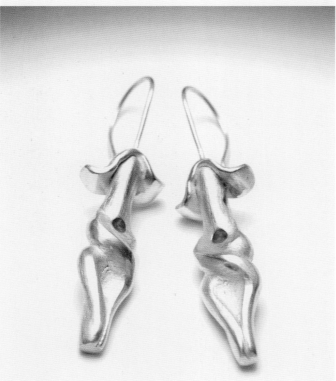

**FRANCE ROY**
Hope for a Miracle

Media: 925 silver, coloured
epoxy resin

Photo: Anthony McLean

**BARBARA CHRISTIE**
GH 40162

Media: 18ct yellow gold, 925 silver,
blue hemimorphites, carved bone

Photo: Barbara Christie

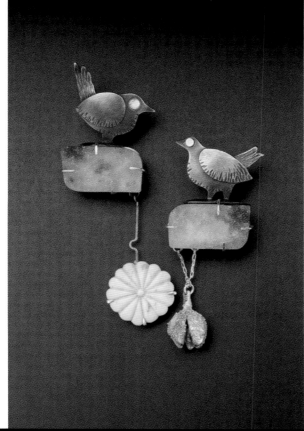

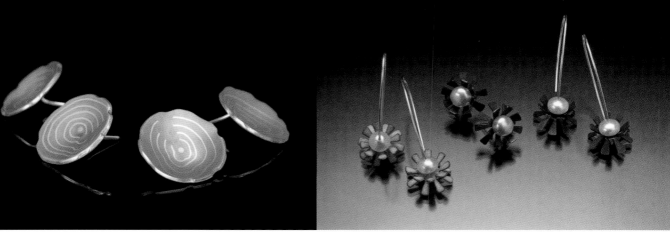

**J. ADRIANNE DIENNO**
Tree Ring Posts

Media: nickel, silver, copper, brass

Photo: Dustin Dienno

**JAN SMITH**
Folded Flower Series

Media: 925 silver, copper, enamel,
pearls, 14ct gold

Photo: Doug Yaple

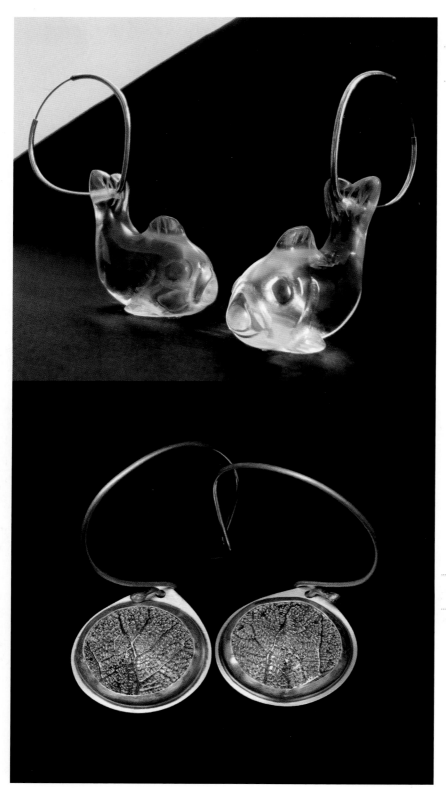

**PACO RIVAS**
Carp

Media: translucent PMMA, silver rings

Photo: Paco Rivas

**SHARON SCHAFFNER**
Tree of Life

Media: 925 silver, electroplated gold

Photo: National Archaeological Museum of Tarragona

**LEONOR HIPÓLITO**
Splendour of Wearability

Medium: silver

Photo: Arne Kaiser

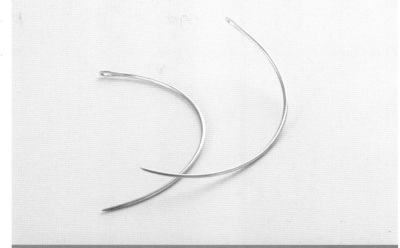

**EMILY WATSON**
Barbell Earrings

Medium: 925 silver

Photo: Emily Watson

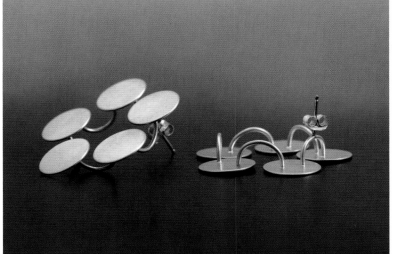

**GERTI MACHACEK**
Red Loop

Media: 925 silver, acrylic glass

Photo: Sophie Pölzl

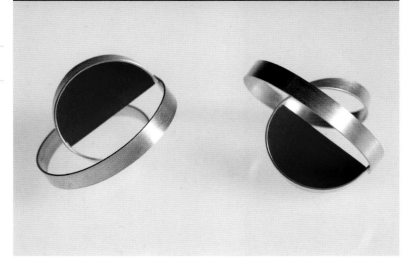

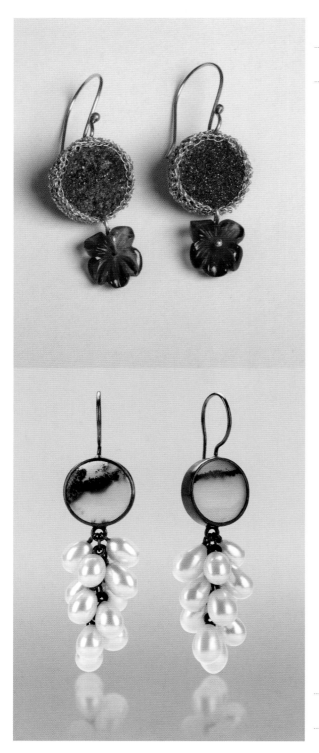

**SU KROKER**
Green Baroque

Media: 18ct gold, uvarovite, amethyst

Photo: Frans Bouwmeester Fotografie

**WALKA STUDIO (Claudia
Betancourt & Nano Pulgar)**
Chains

Media: ox horn, 950 silver

Photo: Karen Clunes

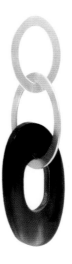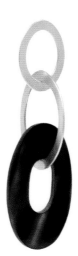

**SENAY AKIN**
Winter Earrings

Media: dendritic agate, freshwater
pearl, 925 silver

Photo: Gokhan Kaya

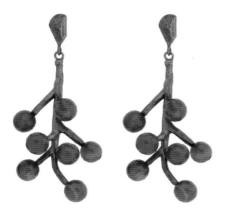

**MARTA CODERQUE**
Raspberry Branches

Media: silver, agate beads

Photo: Coderque Design

**VIKKI KASSIORAS**
Nepheli

Medium: 925 silver

Photo: Terence Bogue

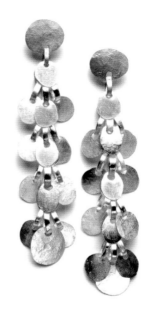

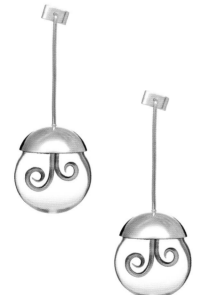

**ELISA PAIVA**
Encapsulated

Media: silver, automotive lamps

Photo: Estudio FM

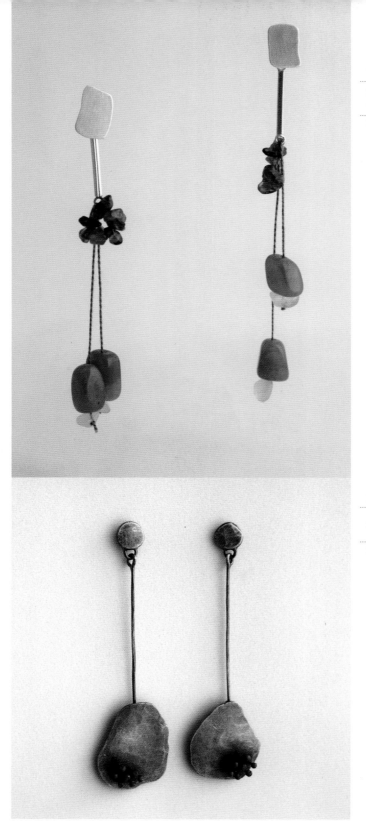

**CUCÚ RUIZ**
Untitled

Media: amethyst, aventurine,
cotton thread, silver

Photo: Cucú Ruiz

**LIISA HASHIMOTO**
Red Moss Earring

Media: silver, red enamel paint

Photo: Liisa Hashimoto

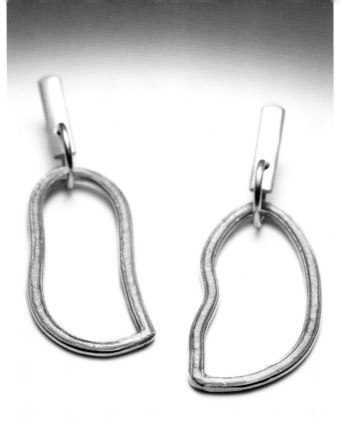

**FRANCE ROY**
Dreams

Media: 925 silver, coloured
epoxy resin

Photo: Anthony McLean

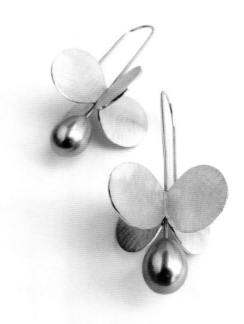

**SENAY AKIN**
Butterfly Earrings

Media: freshwater pearl,
18ct yellow gold, 925 silver

Photo: Senay Akin

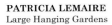

**PATRICIA LEMAIRE**
Large Hanging Gardens

Media: 925 silver, coral

Photo: Ecliptique – Laurent Thion

**AIJA KIVI**
White Flower

........................................................................

Media: silver filigree, freshwater pearl

........................................................................

Photo: Aija Kivi

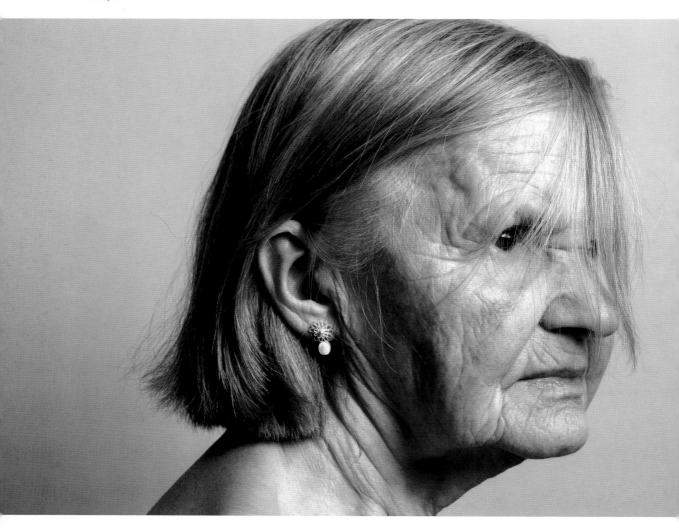

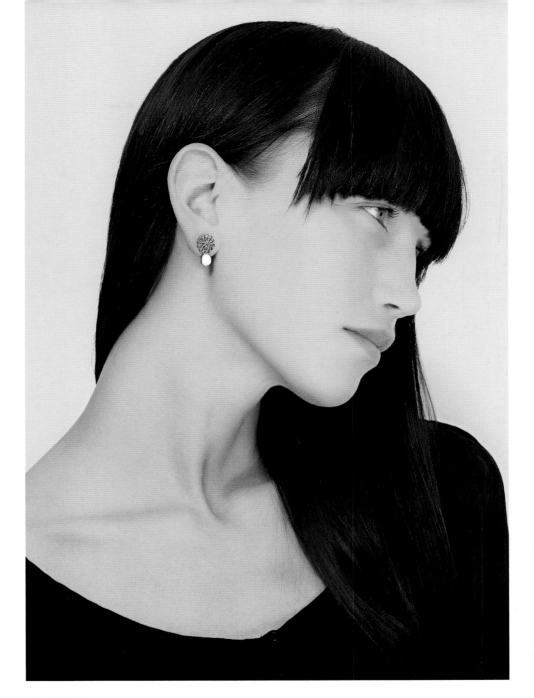

**AIJA KIVI**
Black Flower

Media: silver filigree, freshwater pearl

Photo: Aija Kivi

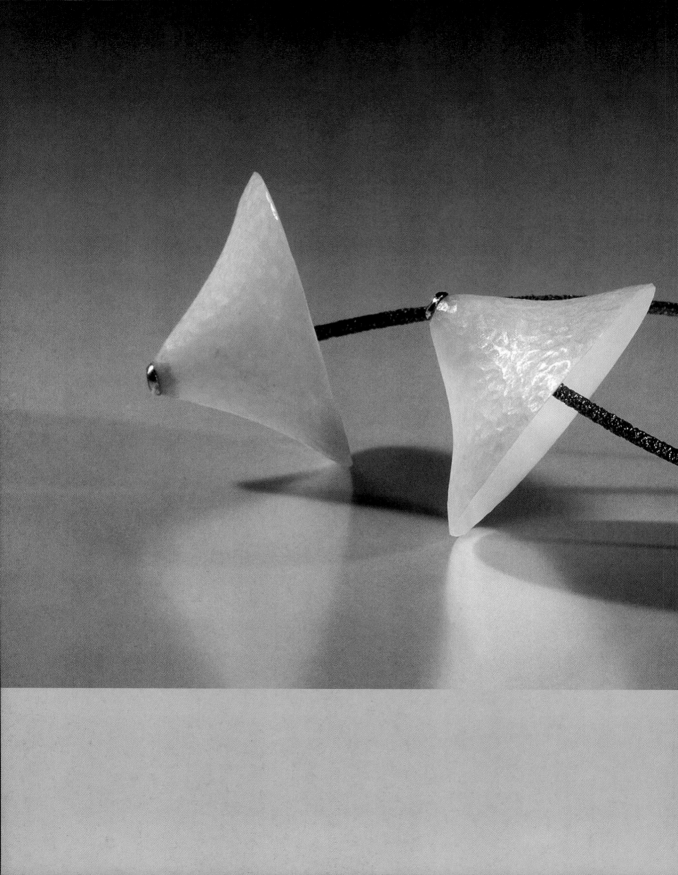

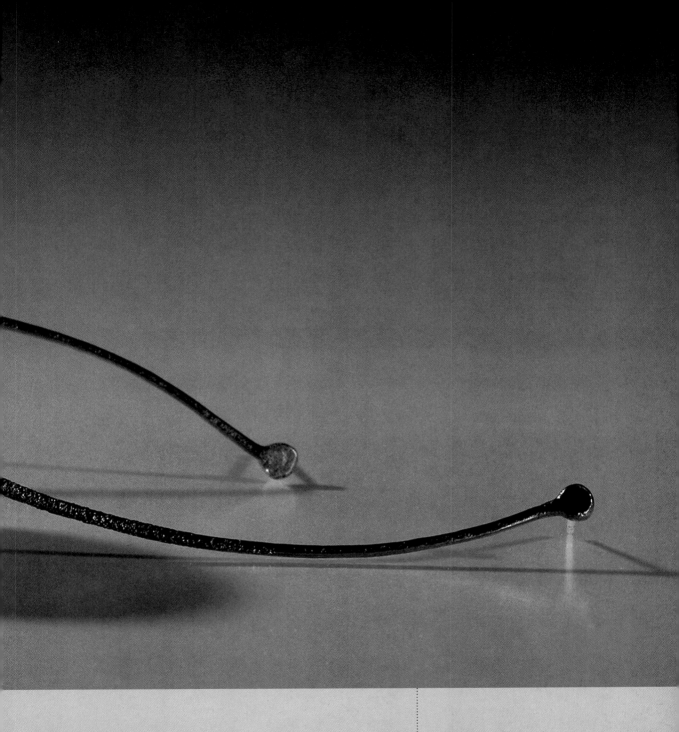

SUBLIME

**JULIA DEVILLE**
Death & Diamonds Earrings

Media: silver, antique rhinestones

Photo: Terence Bogue

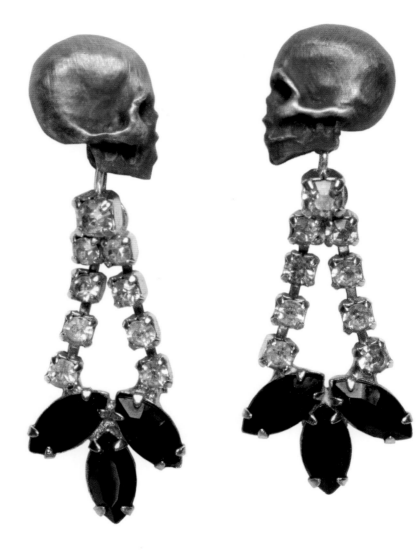

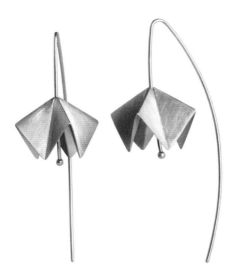

**ANNE BADER**
Calotta

Medium: gold-plated 925 silver

Photo: Stefano Zanini

**ANNE BADER**
Bloom

Medium: 925 silver

Photo: Stefano Zanini

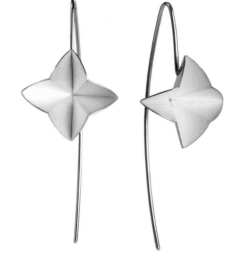

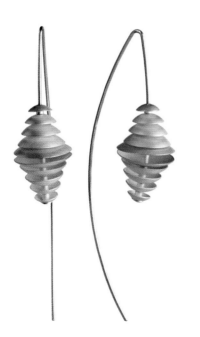

**ANNE BADER**
Settanta

Medium: 925 silver

Photo: Stefano Zanini

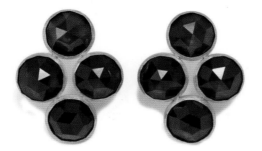

**CHRISTA LÜHTJE**
Untitled

Media: gold, garnet

Photo: Eva Jünger

**BEATE KLOCKMANN**
Untitled

Media: gold, silver, niello

Photo: Beate Klockmann

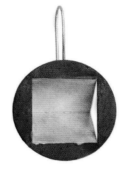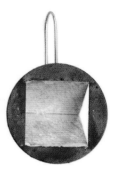

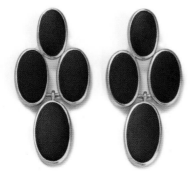

**CHRISTA LÜHTJE**
Untitled

Media: gold, hematite

Photo: Eva Jünger

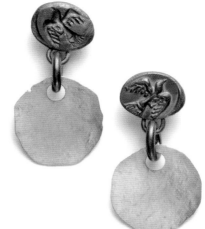

**VIKKI KASSIORAS**
Your Skin will be of Gold

Media: 925 silver, 18ct yellow gold

Photo: Terence Bogue

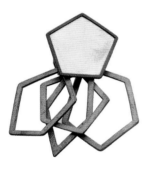 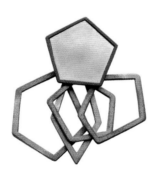

**BABETTE VON DOHNANYI**
Polyps

Media: 925 silver, 18ct gold

Photo: Federico Cavicchioli

**ENRIC MAJORAL**
Chips

Medium: gold

Photo: Majoral

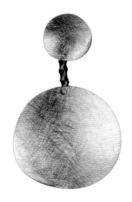 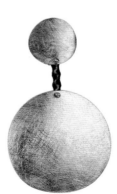

**ANETT JULIANA LEÓN**
Frailejón

Media: 925 silver, 18ct gold

Photo: Anett Juliana León

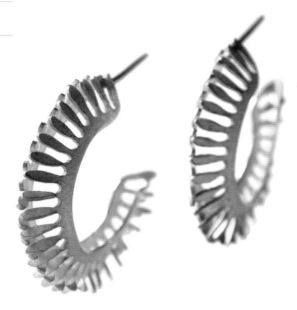

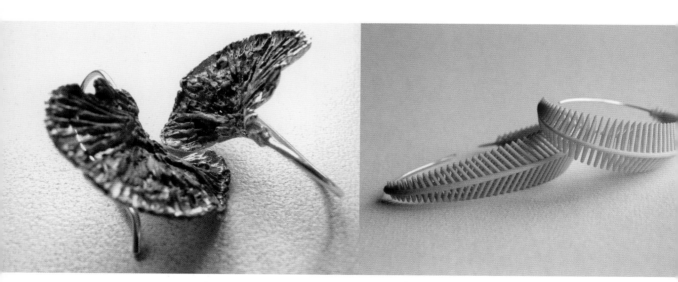

**MARÍA CECILIA GÓMEZ BETANCUR**
Fungus

Media: 925 silver, acrylic paint

Photo: María Cecilia Gómez Betancur

**THERESA BURGER**
Untitled 2011

Media: 3D printed nylon, 925 silver

Photo: Andrew Burger

**LINNÉA ERIKSSON**
Black Gems

Media: steel, silver

Photo: Linnéa Eriksson

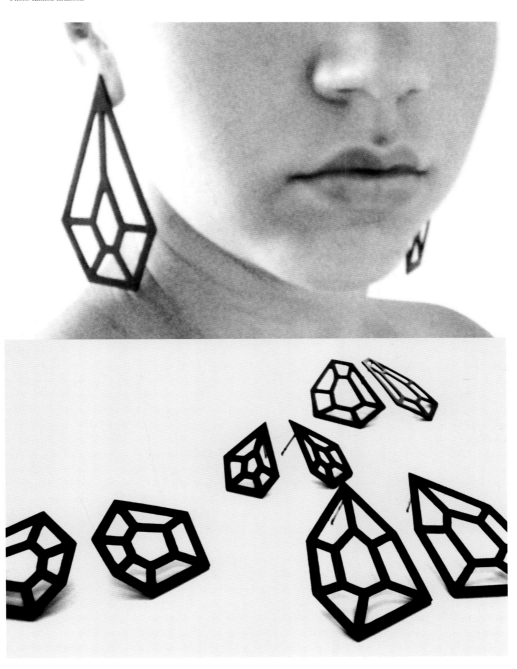

**BEVERLY TADEU**
Rooted Hoops

Media: 18ct gold, silver

Photo: Hap Sakwa

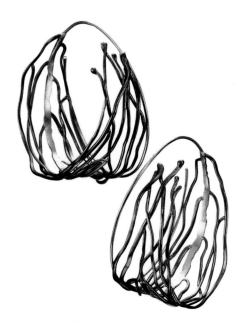

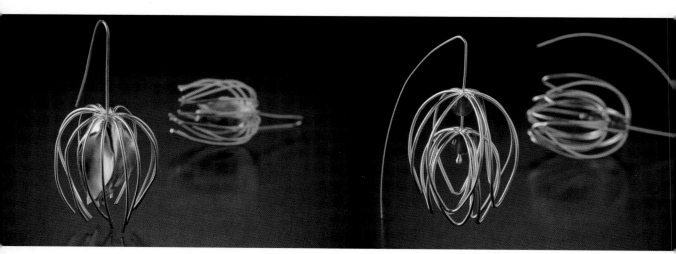

**ALINE KOKINOPOULOS**
Seeds

Media: silver, gold

Photo: Aline Kokinopoulos

**ALINE KOKINOPOULOS**
Physalis

Media: silver, cornelian

Photo: Aline Kokinopoulos

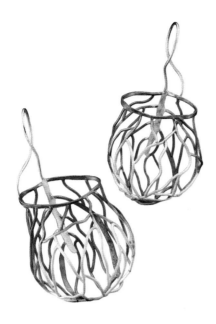

**BEVERLY TADEU**
Rooted Basket

Media: 18ct gold, silver

Photo: Hap Sakwa

**BEVERLY TADEU**
Rooted Hanging

Media: 18ct gold, silver

Photo: Hap Sakwa

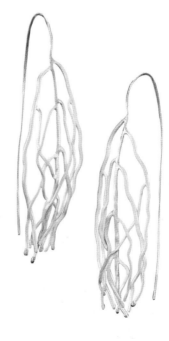

**BEVERLY TADEU**
Mod Pods

Media: 18ct gold, silver

Photo: Hap Sakwa

**PILI ÁNGEL LOSADA**
The Making of Decisions

Medium: 18ct gold

Photo: Adriana Almeida Meza

**PILI ÁNGEL LOSADA**
Metallic Lime Slice Part 2

Media: lime rind, bronze wire,
950 silver, 24ct gold-plated

Photo: Adriana Almeida Meza

**ELVIRA LÓPEZ DEL PRADO**
Blue

Media: enamelled copper wire,
anodized aluminium, glass pebbles,
Swarovski crystal teardrops

Photo: Elvira López del Prado

**ELVIRA LÓPEZ DEL PRADO**
Nile

Media: enamelled copper wire,
cotton threads

Photo: Elvira López del Prado

**ELVIRA LÓPEZ DEL PRADO**
Bulgaria

Media: enamelled copper wire,
anodized aluminium, glass pebbles,
Czech glass beads

Photo: Elvira López del Prado

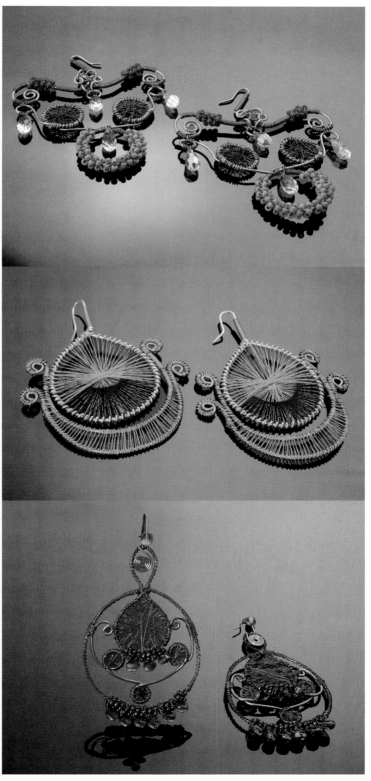

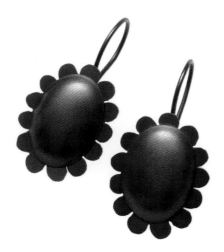

**SIM LUTTIN**
Framed #1

Medium: 925 silver

Photo: Andrew Barcham

**SIM LUTTIN**
Pearl Earrings

Media: 925 silver, freshwater pearl,
18ct gold

Photo: Andrew Barcham

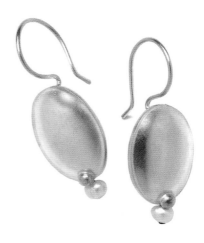

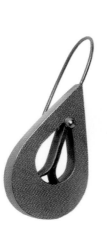
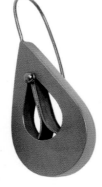

**SIM LUTTIN**
Time Past

Medium: 925 silver

Photo: Andrew Barcham

**JULIA DEVILLE**
Rose Earrings with Onyx Drops

Media: silver, black garnet, onyx

Photo: Terence Bogue

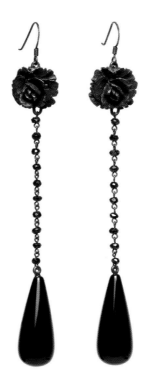

**NICOLE JACQUARD**
Petals

Media: silver, pearl, garnet

Photo: Kevin Montague

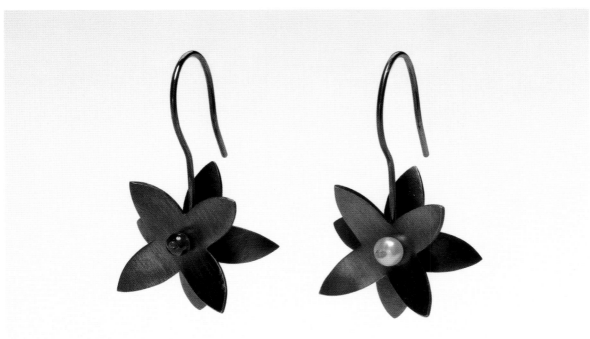

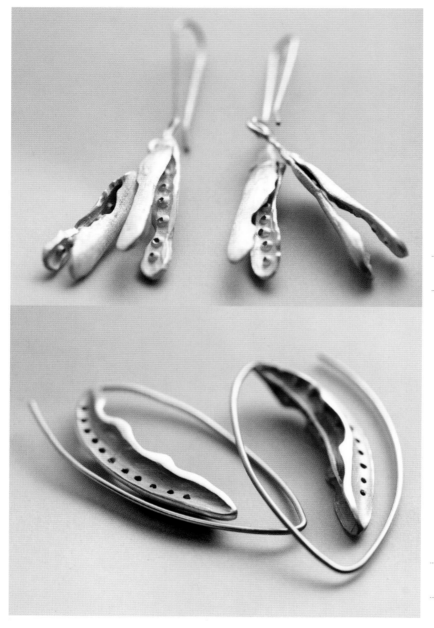

**VÍCTOR SALDARRIAGA**
Qué Vaina

Media: 18ct gold, 950 silver, enamel

Photo: Andrés Gómez

**VÍCTOR SALDARRIAGA**
Qué Vaina

Media: 18ct gold, 950 silver, enamel

Photo: Andrés Gómez

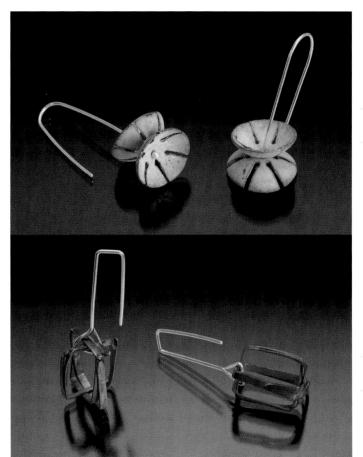

**JAN SMITH**
Enamel Slice Basket

Media: 925 silver, copper, enamel

Photo: Doug Yaple

**JAN SMITH**
Rectangle Basket

Media: 925 silver, 18ct gold

Photo: Doug Yaple

**JAN SMITH**
Basket Weir

Medium: 925 silver

Photo: Doug Yaple

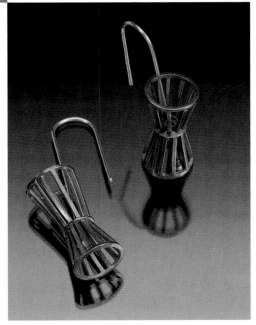

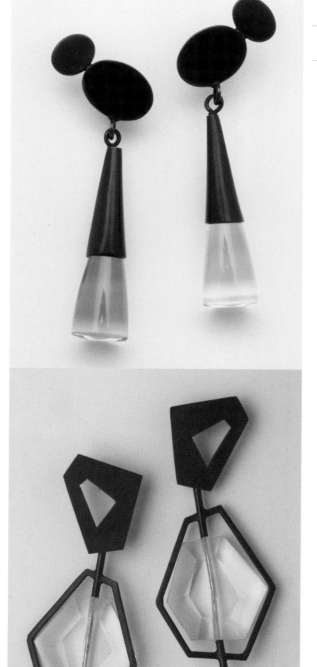

**DAPHNE KRINOS**
Olive Oyl Earrings

Media: silver, citrines

Photo: Joel Degen

**DAPHNE KRINOS**
Earrings

Media: silver, rock crystal

Photo: Joel Degen

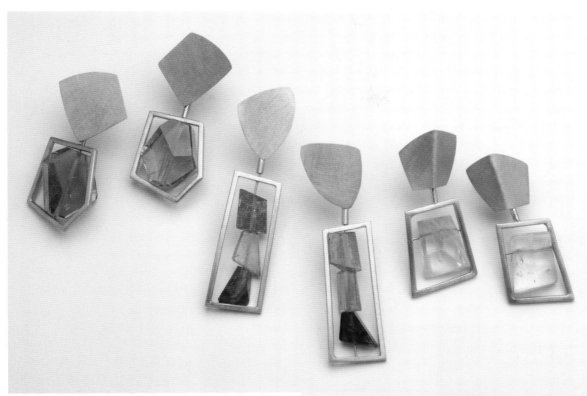

**DAPHNE KRINOS**
Earrings

Media: 18ct gold, citrines,
tourmalines, aquamarines

Photo: Joel Degen

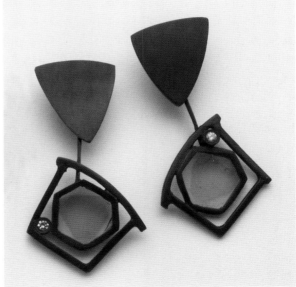

**DAPHNE KRINOS**
Earrings

Media: silver, tourmalines,
diamonds

Photo: Joel Degen

**ADRIANA HENAO MEJÍA**
Heliconia –
The Enchanted Garden

Medium: 950 silver

Photo: Jorge Mario Múnera

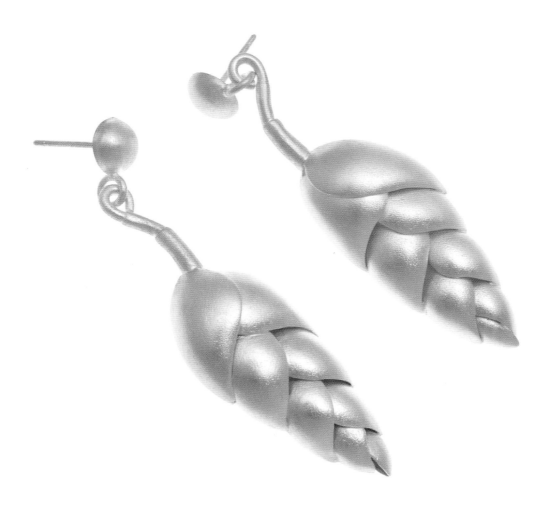

**FRÉDÉRIQUE COOMANS**
Squamate Earrings I

Media: PMMA, metallic effect
polyester thread

Photo: Anne-Lise Chopin

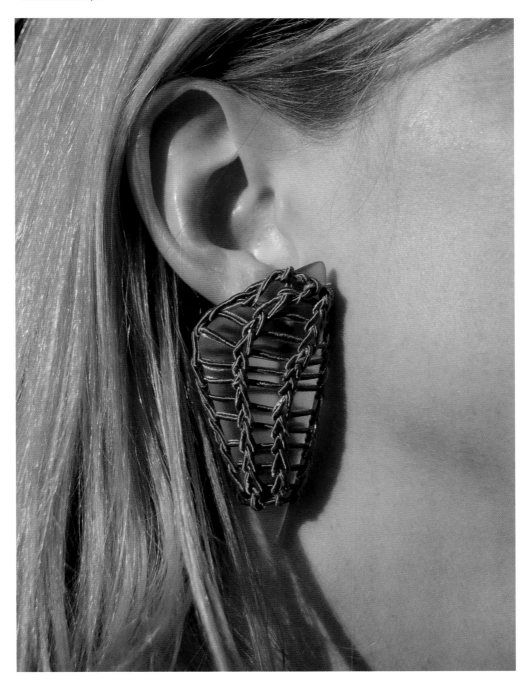

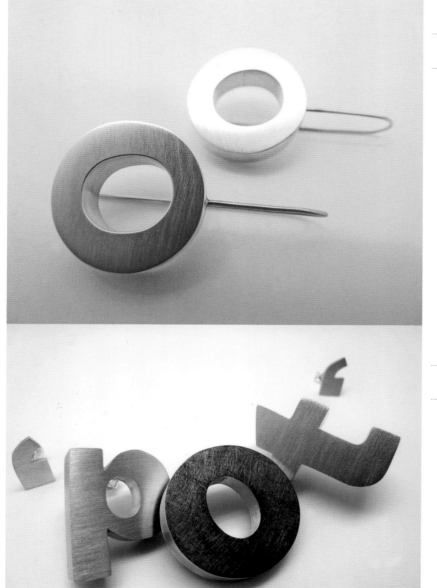

**IÑAKI SALOM**
Chunky Silver 'O' Earrings
with Hooks – Typo Collection

Medium: 925 silver

Photo: Iñaki Salom

**IÑAKI SALOM**
Chunky Silver and Gold
Earrings – Typo Collection

Media: 925 silver, 18ct gold

Photo: Iñaki Salom

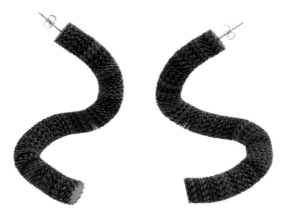

**JENNACA DAVIES**
Paper Spiral Earrings

Media: laser-cut paper, 925 silver

Photo: Steffen Knudsen Allen

**NICOLE JACQUARD**
Ruby Clips

Media: silver, rubies, monofilament

Photo: Kevin Montague

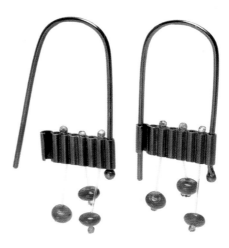

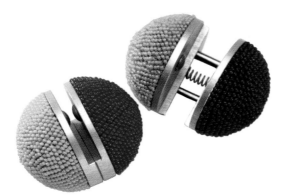

**JACQUELINE I. LILLIE**
Clip-on Earrings

Media: aluminium, glass beads

Photo: Uli Kohl

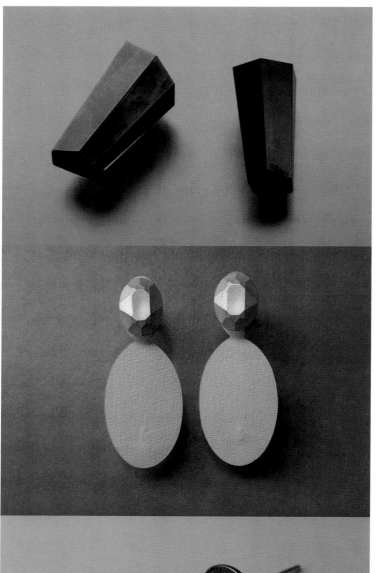

**BABETTE VON DOHNANYI**
Crystal Earrings

Media: 925 silver, jet

Photo: Federico Cavicchioli

**BLANCA SÁNCHEZ**
Untitled – Brilliant Collection

Medium: silver

Photo: Blanca Sánchez

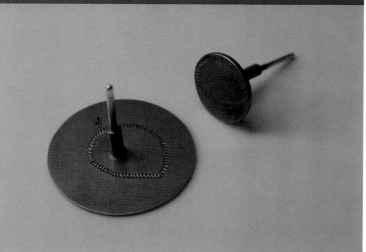

**BLANCA SÁNCHEZ**
Untitled

Medium: silver

Photo: Blanca Sánchez

**CONSTANZA SOTO DONOSO**
Copper Cells

Media: copper, sheep's wool

Photo: Constanza Soto Donoso

**RYAN DE JAGER**
Blossoms

Media: 925 silver, plastic

Photo: Ryan de Jager

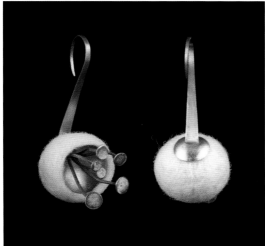

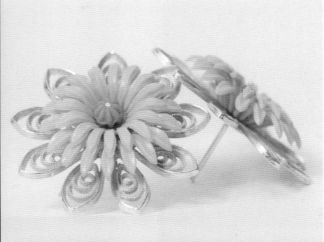

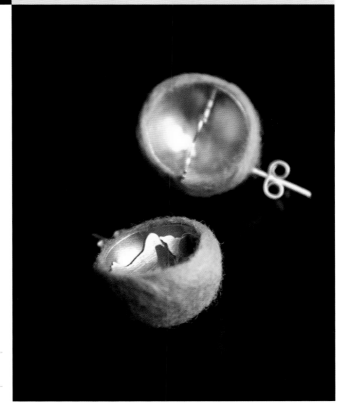

**CONSTANZA SOTO DONOSO**
Pigeon's Nests

Media: 925 silver, sheep's wool

Photo: Constanza Soto Donoso

**ULLA & MARTIN KAUFMANN**
Folded

Medium: 18ct gold

Photo: M. Hoffmann

**ULLA & MARTIN KAUFMANN**
In the Circle

Medium: 18ct gold

Photo: H.P. Hoffmann

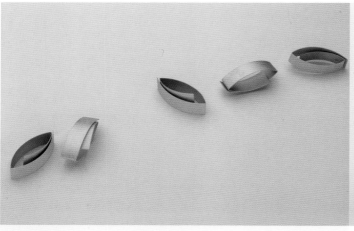

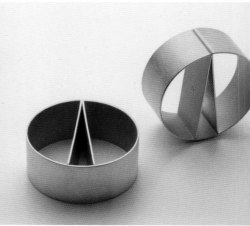

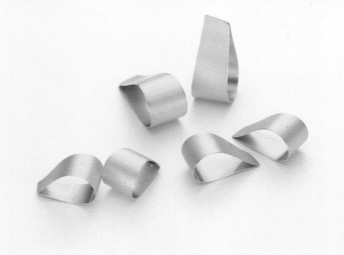

**ULLA & MARTIN KAUFMANN**
Loop

Medium: 18ct gold

Photo: M. Hoffmann

## SÒNIA SERRANO
Translucent 3

Media: epoxy resin, silver

Photo: Sònia Serrano

## SÒNIA SERRANO
Translucent 2

Media: epoxy resin, silver

Photo: Sònia Serrano

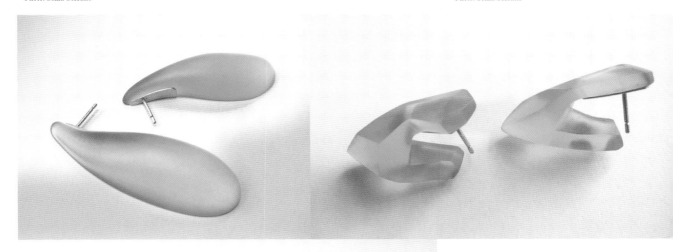

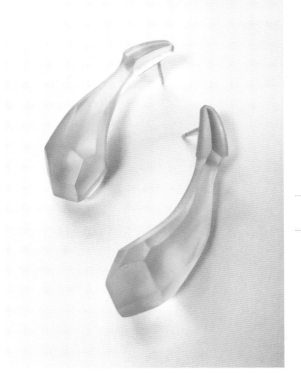

## SÒNIA SERRANO
Translucent 1

Media: epoxy resin, silver

Photo: Sònia Serrano

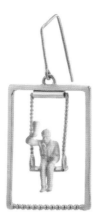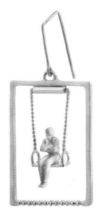

**YAEL SERFATY & TAL SALOMON**
Frame 3

Media: silver, white resin figures

Photo: Hadass Blankistain

**YAEL SERFATY & TAL SALOMON**
Royal Garden

Media: silver, white resin figures

Photo: Hadass Blankistain

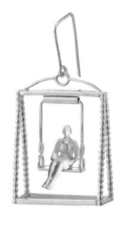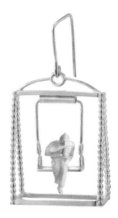

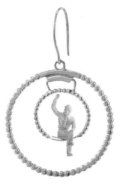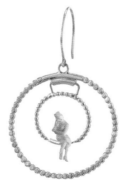

**YAEL SERFATY & TAL SALOMON**
Swing on a Star

Media: silver, white resin figures

Photo: Hadass Blankistain

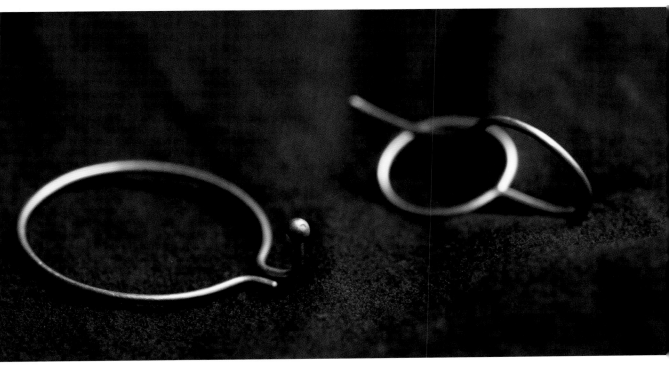

**SALVADOR MALLOL**
Ora / Vuit Earrings

Media: yellow gold, white gold

Photo: Didac Cirera – Fotomaton

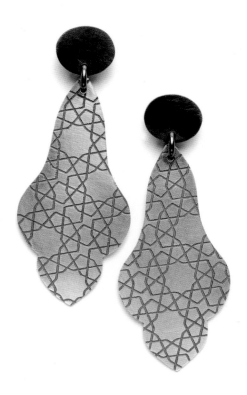

**VIKKI KASSIORAS**
Arabia

Media: 925 silver, computer engraved
Arabic geometric pattern

Photo: Terence Bogue

**ROC MAJORAL & ABRIL RIBERA**
Butterfly

Medium: silver

Photo: Majoral

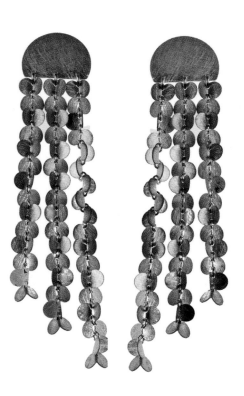

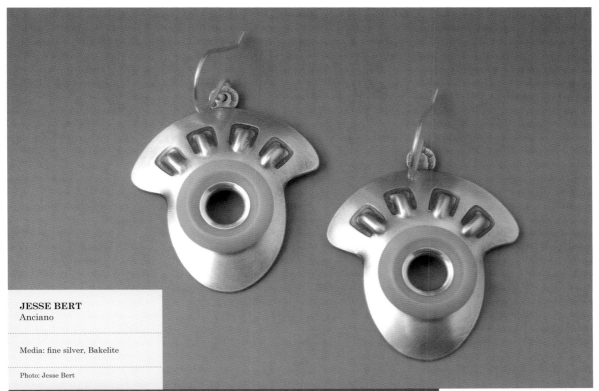

**JESSE BERT**
Anciano

Media: fine silver, Bakelite

Photo: Jesse Bert

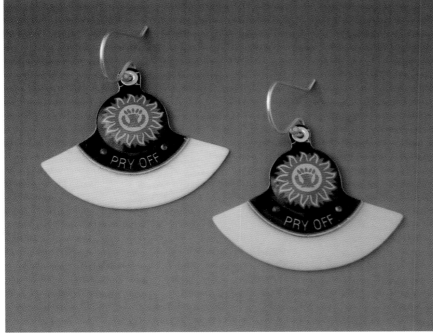

**JESSE BERT**
Pry Off

Media: silver, ivory recycled from
antique piano keys, bottle caps,
copper

Photo: Jesse Bert

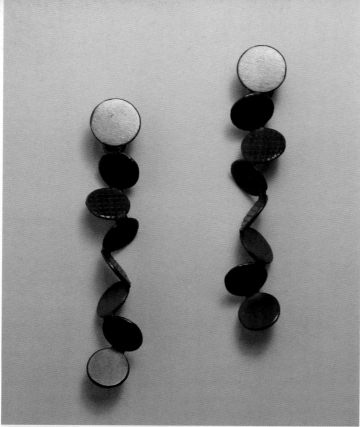

**MISUN WON**
Simple Dangling Earrings

Media: 925 silver, keum-boo,
24ct gold foil

Photo: Misun Won

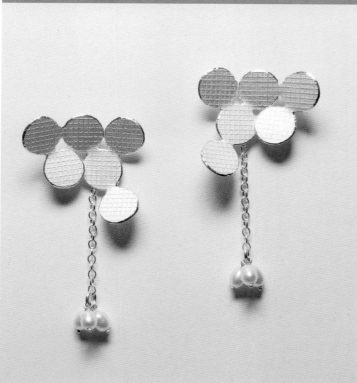

**MISUN WON**
Six Circles Earrings with Pearl

Media: 925 silver, pearl

Photo: Misun Won

**EMILY WATSON**
Cellulose Earrings

Media: 925 silver, dyed wood

Photo: Emily Watson

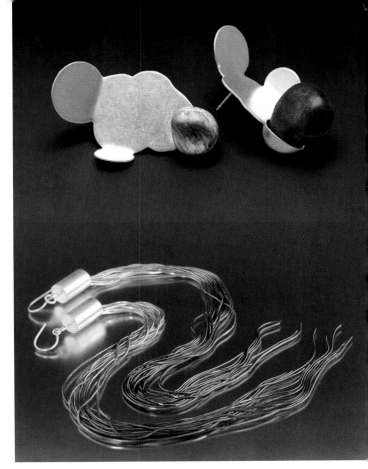

**L. SUE SZABO**
Foot-Long Earrings

Medium: 925 silver

Photo: Katy Mims

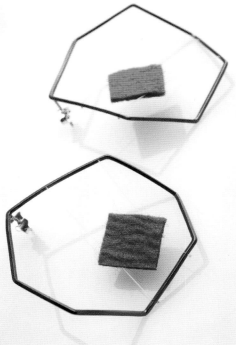

**IRO KASKANI**
Why Not?

Media: 925 silver, plastic cord, felt

Photo: Dimitris Vattis

**ANNE BADER**
Medusa

Medium: 925 silver

Photo: Stefano Zanini

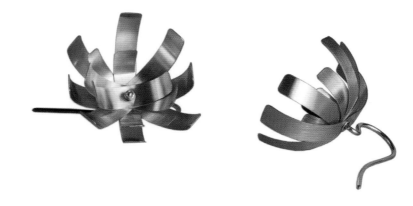

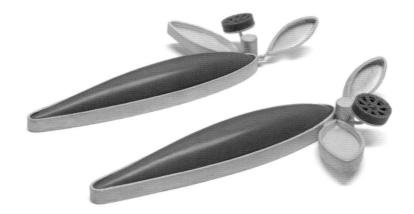

**KATJA PRINS**
Flowerpiece Earrings

Media: silver, plastic

Photo: Francis Willemstijn

## ENRIC MAJORAL
Exclusive Piece

Media: gold, imperial topaz

Photo: Majoral

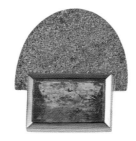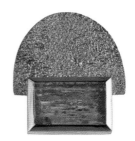

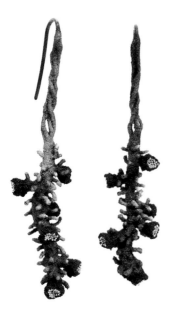

## ARATA FUCHI
Nostalgia 4

Media: 950 silver, silver powder,
fine gold

Photo: Arata Fuchi

## ANNE BADER
Piega

Medium: gold-plated 925 silver

Photo: Stefano Zanini

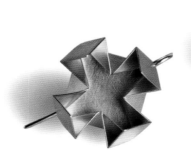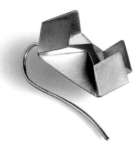

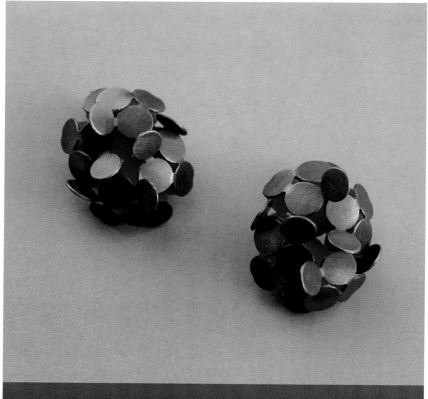

**MISUN WON**
Oval Wrapping Earrings

Media: 925 silver, orange
enamel paint

Photo: Misun Won

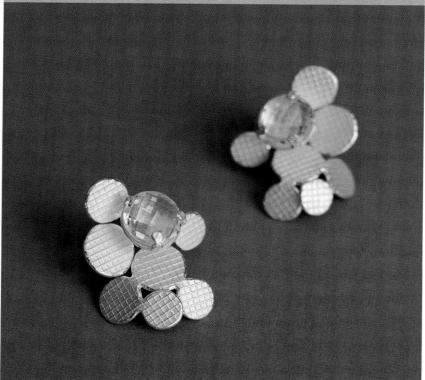

**MISUN WON**
Random Pattern with
Rock Crystal Earrings

Media: 925 silver, rock crystal

Photo: Misun Won

**GERTI MACHACEK**
Flower Fish

Medium: 925 silver

Photo: Sophie Pölzl

**GERTI MACHACEK**
Fish Flower

Medium: 925 silver

Photo: Sophie Pölzl

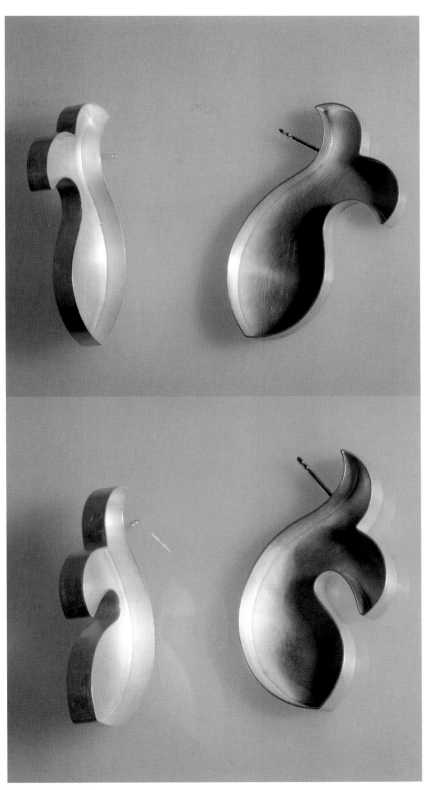

## L. SUE SZABO
Colour Me Up

Media: enamel on copper,
925 silver, steel cable

Photo: Ericka Crissman

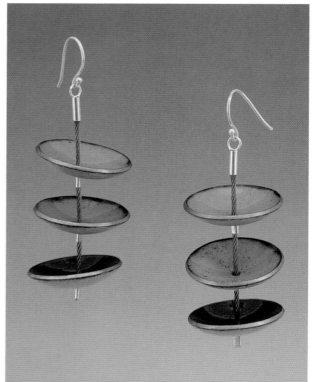

## JESSE BERT
Switch Button

Media: copper, fine silver, ivory from
antique piano keys, antique copper,
ebony

Photo: Jesse Bert

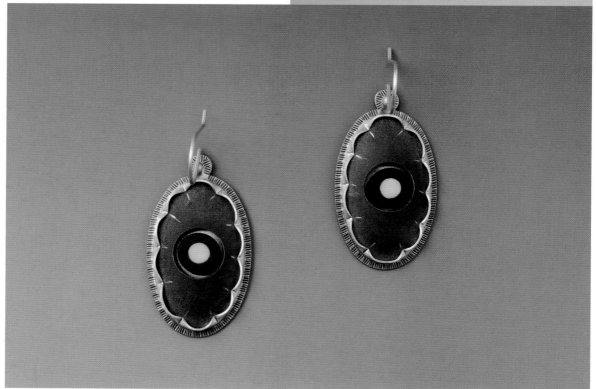

**DENISE QUEIROZ**
Joy

Media: 18ct white gold, rubellite,
diamonds

Photo: Marcos Vianna

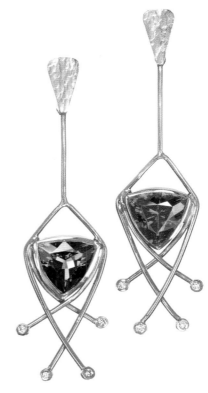

**LIAUNG-CHUNG YEN**
Flourishing Series #12

Media: 22ct and 18ct gold,
925 silver

Photo: Liaung-Chung Yen

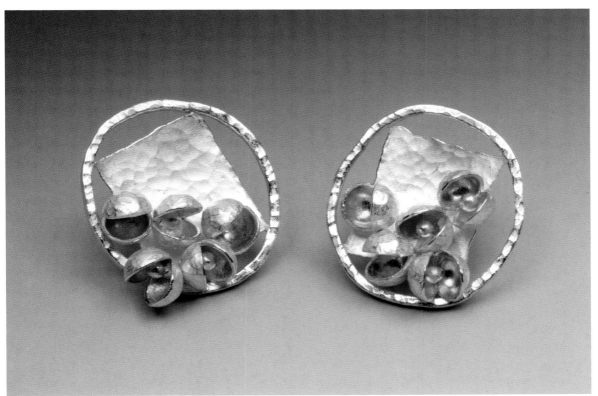

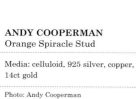

**ANDY COOPERMAN**
Orange Spiracle Stud

Media: celluloid, 925 silver, copper,
14ct gold

Photo: Andy Cooperman

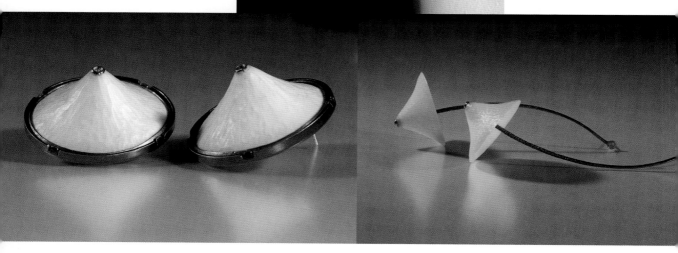

**ANDY COOPERMAN**
White Spiracle Studs

Media: celluloid, 925 silver, copper,
bronze, 14ct gold

Photo: Andy Cooperman

**ANDY COOPERMAN**
Orange Parasols

Media: celluloid, 925 silver, copper,
14ct gold

Photo: Andy Cooperman

**COLLECTIVE FALABRAC**
Millebolle

Medium: 925 silver

Photo: Falabrac

**COLLECTIVE FALABRAC**
Millebolle

Media: white techno-nylon, silver

Photo: Falabrac

**COLLECTIVE FALABRAC**
Millebolle

Media: black techno-nylon, gold

Photo: Falabrac

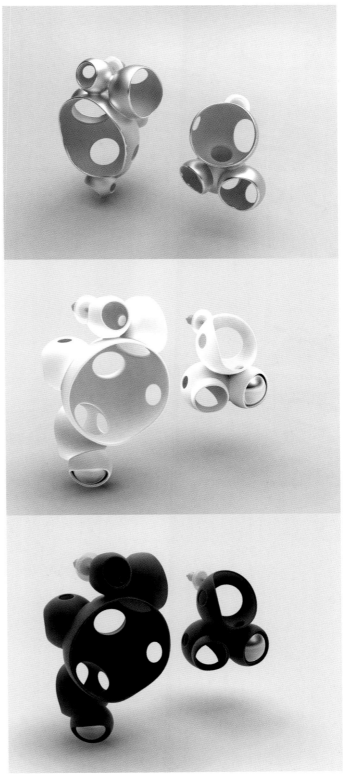

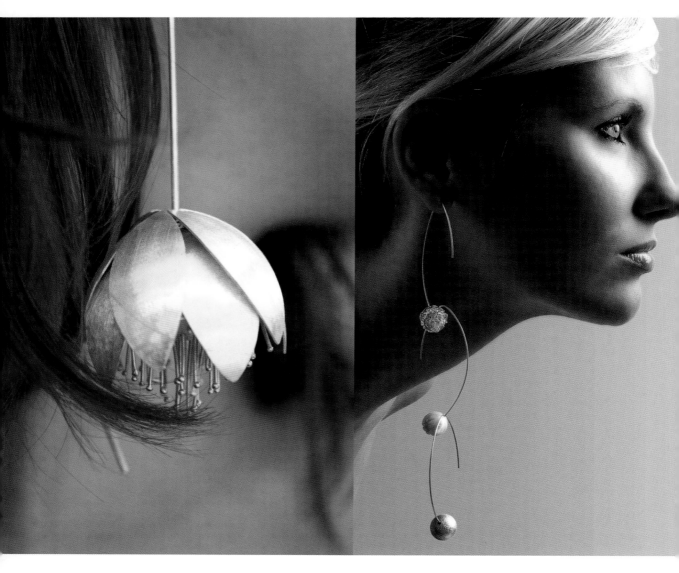

**AINA MINISTRAL**
Lotus Flower

Media: silver, gold-plated silver

Photo: Agnés Mora

**TIFFANY ROWE**
Recto Verso

Media: silver, metal wire, white coral

Photo: Geoffroy Baud

**ANTJE STOLZ**
As Light as a Stone I

Media: slate veneer, enamel paint,
14ct gold

Photo: Antje Stolz

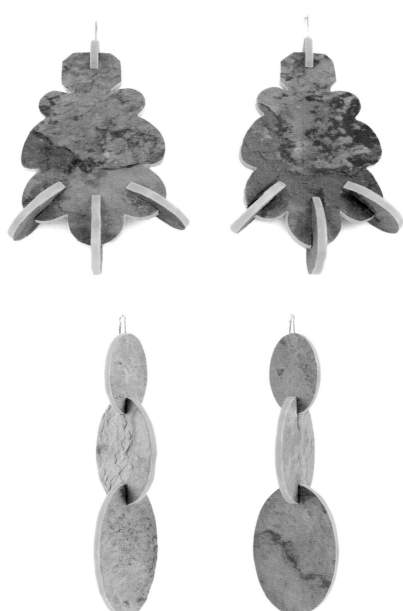

**ANTJE STOLZ**
As Light as a Stone II

Media: slate veneer, enamel paint,
14ct gold

Photo: Antje Stolz

**DANIEL DICAPRIO**
Vitae Earrings

Media: lignum vitae, 22ct gold

Photo: Daniel DiCaprio

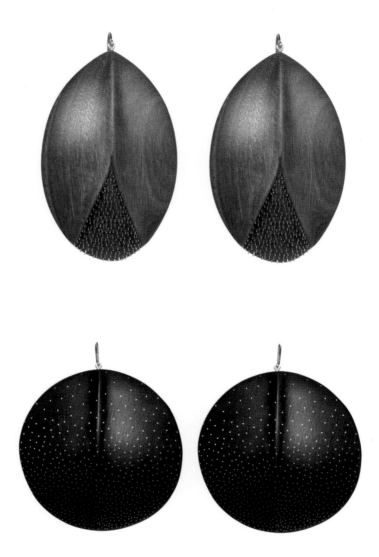

**DANIEL DICAPRIO**
Disc Earrings

Media: ebony, silver

Photo: Daniel DiCaprio

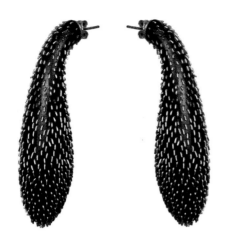

**DANIEL DICAPRIO**
Droplet Earrings 2

Media: ebony, silver

Photo: Daniel DiCaprio

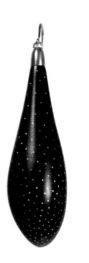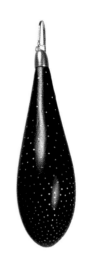

**DANIEL DICAPRIO**
Droplet Earrings

Media: ebony, silver

Photo: Daniel DiCaprio

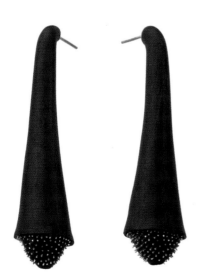

**DANIEL DICAPRIO**
New Growth Earrings

Media: ebony, 22ct gold

Photo: Daniel DiCaprio

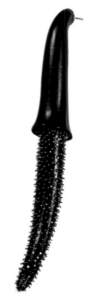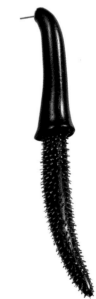

**DANIEL DICAPRIO**
Emerge Earrings

Media: ebony, silver

Photo: Daniel DiCaprio

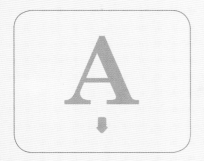

## ADRIANA HENAO MEJÍA
Colombian
*aurea@aureajoyas.com | www.aureajoyas.com*
Boasting over fifteen years' experience, Medellín-born designer Adriana Henao Mejía's training combines self-study with courses in enamelling, embossing, keum-boo, engraving and lost-wax casting. Seeking to demonstrate the value of jewelry beyond its economic worth, Adriana combines the traditional and the contemporary within her work. Delighting in the creative process, she explores themes such as nature, ethnic American iconography, ancient cultures and dreams. She has been featured in numerous exhibitions, both in Colombia and abroad, and in books including *New Rings: 500+ Designs from Around the World.* > pp. 86, 134, 198, 199

## AIJA KIVI
Estonian
*aija.kivi@hotmail.com*
*www.aijakivi.com*
*aijakivi.blogspot.com*
Aija Kivi pursued her studies in jewelry-making at the Estonian Academy of Arts, in the capital city of Tallinn. Her pieces above all emphasize delicacy and beauty, a concern powerfully symbolized for the artist by the leaves of dried flowers, whose fragile allure she endeavours to capture by finding the balance between complexity and simplicity. In late 2011 she held a solo exhibition of her work at the A-Galerii in central Tallinn. > pp. 178, 179

## AINA MINISTRAL
Spanish
*ainajoies@gmail.com*
Up-and-coming Barcelona-born designer Aina Ministral employs natural stones and precious metals to convey the harmony and simplicity of natural forms. Despite her young age, she has completed extensive training, apprenticing at the Centre d'Art La Rectoria and attending practical workshops and courses at the likes of the Massana School, dterra and the Catalan Federation of Jewelers, Goldsmiths and Watchmakers (JORGC), whom she represented in the 2009 exhibition 'L'Estellera'. She is certified by the University of Barcelona and the Federation of European Education in Gemmology. > pp. 20, 224

## ALEXIS KOSTUK
Canadian
*alexis.glaciale@gmail.com*
*glacialegoldsmith.blogspot.com*
Having developed an interest in jewelry while studying at Toronto's OCAD University, Alexis Kostuk furthered her education with a one-year intensive course at the Istituto Europeo di Design in Milan, Italy. Since returning to Toronto, she has combined producing her own pieces under the name Glaciale with managing local cooperative studio Jewel Envy. Often mixing different artistic media, Alexis especially relishes experimenting with alternative materials and using metals intuitively. She is fascinated by the relationship between people, objects and memories. > pp. 45, 66

## ALINE KOKINOPOULOS
Senegalese
*alinek67@yahoo.fr | alinek.jimdo.com*
Born in Senegal in 1967, Aline Kokinopoulos studied jewelry-making in Vitrolles and Nimes under Gilles Jonemann and Joël Faivre-Chalon respectively, as well as undertaking workshops with Tasso Mattar and Esther Brinkmann. Now boasting over twenty years' experience, she embeds imagery from dreams, nature and her surroundings into her creations, which are chiefly worked in silver and stones. In addition to recent exhibitions in Paris, Livorno and Padua, her work is showcased in books including *1000 Rings* and *The Compendium Finale of Contemporary Jewellers.* > pp. 21, 159, 188

## AMY TAVERN
American
*amy@amytavern.com | www.amytavern.com*
*amytavern.blogspot.com*
The holder of a BFA from the University of Washington, Amy Tavern has exhibited domestically at Velvet da Vinci and Sienna Gallery and abroad at Beyond Fashion, in Antwerp, Belgium. Her designs have been reproduced in the books *500 Silver Jewelry Designs* and *New Rings* and in *Metalsmith* magazine. Amy's unique pieces combine varied influences such as antique jewelry and graffiti. The winner of the 2009 American Craft Council Searchlight Artist Award, she is currently a resident artist at North Carolina's Penland School of Crafts. > pp. 80, 83, 88

## ANA MARÍA RAMÍREZ MOURE
Colombian
*ana_mmoure@yahoo.es*
*anacuaderno.blogspot.com*
*cuadernobandada.blogspot.com*
Ana María Ramírez Moure was born in Bogotá, Colombia, where she completed an undergraduate degree in fine art, specializing in sculpture. After moving to Barcelona in 2000, she began designing her own jewelry while consolidating her education at the Massana and Elisava Schools respectively. She has taken her work, which is influenced by organic forms, to exhibitions in Bogotá, Paris, Barcelona and San Francisco, as well as contributing to books such as *New Rings*. She is also one half of the jewelry/industrial design project Bandada. > p. 46

## ALEXIS KOSTUK (ANDRA OANA LUPU)
ANDRA OANA LUPU
Romanian
*contact@andralupu.com | andralupu.com*
After completing undergraduate design studies at the University of Art and Design in her birthplace of Cluj-Napoca, Romania, Andra Oana Lupu stayed on to study for a PhD in contemporary jewelry. Her distinctly experimental, eclectic and unconventional work is driven by an observation of the development of jewelry and art objects in relation to social and cultural contexts. She has taken part in exhibitions in her hometown and both domestic and international contests, including the 'Dining in 2015' competition, run by prestigious online design magazine *designboom.* > p. 87

## ANDREA CODERCH VALOR
Spanish
*www.andreacoderch.com*
Andrea Coderch Valor undertook her undergraduate studies in industrial design in her hometown of Alcoy, near Alicante. However, she has enjoyed numerous stints abroad, including an Erasmus exchange in Elgin, Scotland, a Promoe grant in Aguascalientes, Mexico, and a five-month stay in London. She subsequently moved to Florence, Italy, studying at the Alchimia School and completing a Leonardo da Vinci work placement in jewelry packaging. Her exhibition experience includes a solo showcase at JOYA 2011 in Barcelona. > p. 123

## ANDREA VELÁZQUEZ CALLEJA
Spanish
*andreavelazquez@tiny-lab.com*
*www.tiny-lab.com*
*andreavelazquez.blogspot.com*
After learning her trade at Barcelona's Massana School and Industrial School, Andrea Velázquez Calleja was named first runner-up at the 2011 Enjoia't Competition and has exhibited in Barcelona at Massana, the Poble Espanyol and FAD (Fostering Arts and Design). Andrea has completed courses in techniques as diverse as lost-wax and primitive casting, keum-boo, ceramics, Berber jewelry and enamelling. Marketing her work under her brand Tiny, she experiments with these methods in her pieces, which aim to make people look and feel beautiful. > p. 135

## ANDY COOPERMAN
American
*andy@andycooperman.com*
*andycooperman.com*
A graduate of the State University of New York College at Oneonta, Andy Cooperman has been a full-time metalsmith since 1987. His work explores particular materials, experiences or points of view through ideas that seize his attention. Andy's exhibition highlights include the 2011 solo show 'Esoterica: Through the Looking Glass' at the Memphis-based National Ornamental Metal Museum and 'Metalsmiths Linking: A Crosscultural Exchange' in Tokyo, Japan. Book features range from *The Penland Book of Jewelry* to both volumes of *Art Jewelry Today.* > p. 222

# INDEX OF ARTISTS

## ANETT JULIANA LEÓN
Colombian
*leonj82@gmail.com*
Anett León has completed copious training and earned numerous official qualifications and awards in her native Colombia. Having been invited to take part in the 2010 'Kilates de Amor' exhibition, in the same year she won a Young Talent Scholarship from the Colombian Institute of Educational Credit and Technical Studies Abroad (ICETEX), allowing her to pursue studies in Barcelona, Spain. Her elegant, expressive pieces draw on a palette of traditional Colombian handicrafts and techniques, which she explores through the lens of nature. > p. 186

## ANGELA BUBASH
American
*angelabubash@gmail.com*
*www.angelabubash.com*
Studio artist and experienced jewelry teacher Angela Bubash has earned grants from the Ruth and Harold Chenven Foundation, the North Carolina Arts Council and the Ludwig Vogelstein Foundation and a residency at Penland School of Crafts. Her work has adorned galleries in the US and Quebec, Canada, and books such as *500 Metal Vessels*, *500 Earrings* and *The Art & Craft of Making Jewelry*. Combining a healthy respect for tradition with contemporary awareness, Angela's pieces invite personal contemplation, capture fleeting emotions and turn experiences into material reality.
> pp. 47, 149

## ANGELO VERGA
Italian
*info@angeloverga.com*
*www.angeloverga.com*
Angelo Verga studied at the State Arts School in Brera, Milan. Boasting over ten years' experience, his work has travelled to exhibitions including the 2011 shows 'Pedrocchi' in Padua and 'Ring Party' in Senigallia, both in Italy, as well as appearing in *New Rings*, published in the same year. Angelo's mixed-media pieces engage in the act of balancing man-made and natural forms, fusing industrial materials, precious metals and mokume gane with the likes of wood. This process is perfectly embodied in his 'Sintered Nature' series.
> p. 86

## ANNE BADER
German
*auri.info@googlemail.com*
*www.auri-jewellery.com*
A native and resident of Giessen, central Germany, Anne Bader qualified as a goldsmith at the nearby Hanau Academy of Drawing. Alongside shows in her home country in Hanover and Dusseldorf, she exhibited in Rome in both 2010 and 2011. Designed under the brand Auri Jewellery, Anne's creations are seemingly weightless, creating an illusion of movement. They consist of thin gold and silver sheets that are layered, sequenced, ordered and even folded like origami.
> pp. 167, 183, 199, 216, 217

## ANNE PERBET JACKSON
French
*aperbet@yahoo.fr*
*anneperbet.canalblog.com*
Paris-born artist Anne Perbet Jackson began her career as a ceramicist. However, after a one-year stint in London, she fell in love with Switzerland, studying in Geneva and settling in Vevey. Her work has been showcased repeatedly across Switzerland and in Swiss publications such as *L'Illustré* and *24heures*. Anne's inventive jewelry synthesizes her miscellaneous experiences, inspiring people to dream. Her nostalgic memories of the seaside and shell-collecting led to her frequent use of porcelain, whose name originally derives from the Italian word for a cowrie shell. > p. 150

## ANNIE TUNG
Canadian
*she.smiled.and.ran@gmail.com*
*www.shesmiledandran.com*
An OCAD University graduate who won the 2010 Toronto Outdoor Art Exhibition's Best of Show in the Sculpture category, Vancouver-born Annie Tung has graced books such as *New Rings*, *500 Plastic Jewelry Designs* and *500 Wedding Rings* and exhibitions including the Silver Triennial 2010 and the 2011 Cheongju International Craft Biennale. Her unconventional, unsettling and poetic work relentlessly explores the links between mortality, time, function, ornament, desire and absence. It is influenced by Victorian memorial practices, the Japanese concept of *wabi-sabi* and the memento mori tradition. > p. 38

## ANTJE STOLZ
German
*antje@stolzesdesign.com* | *www.stolzesdesign.com*
After pursuing classical goldsmithing, Antje Stolz learned gemstone and jewelry design in Idar-Oberstein, Germany and at the Estonian Academy of Arts, Tallinn. The winner of the First Prize in the German Young Talent Competition for Gemstone & Jewellery Design, her work has been displayed at the Marzee Gallery in the Netherlands, SOFA New York, the International Jewellery Competition in Legnica, Poland, and publications such as 2011's *SchmuckDenken/ThinkingJewellery*. Antje's playful pieces manipulate cut stones through the use of contours, engravings, cut-outs and imprints, juxtaposing perception, illusion and associations. > pp. 34, 88, 225

## ARATA FUCHI
Japanese
*mail@arata-fuchi.com* | *www.arata-fuchi.com*
An industrial design graduate from Tokyo Zokei University, Arata Fuchi moved to Florence, Italy, to attend the prestigious Le Arti Orafe jewelry school. She has contributed to exhibitions from New York to Munich and publications including *New Rings*, the *Contemporary Jewellery Yearbook 2011* and *Dreaming Jewelry*. A multi-award-winner (including the BKV-Prize and the Mario Pinton International Award), Arata Fuchi creates her own distinctive take on the Japanese sense of beauty with her 'pulverization' technique, melding the vitality of nature, keum-boo and an expressionist sense of form. > p. 217

## ÅSA ELMSTAM
Swedish
*info@asaelmstam.se*
*www.asaelmstam.se*
At once an artist, product designer and silversmith, Åsa Elmstam utilizes art as a medium to lobby for change and express her dissatisfaction with the current state of affairs. A notable example comes with the borrowing of images from cattle-rearing to explore the trend for mass production and consumption. Åsa followed up an undergraduate metal design degree in her native Sweden, where she has exhibited on numerous occasions, with graduate studies at Tokyo Zokei University. Her work has been featured in several European magazines. > p. 124

## AURELIE DELLASANTA
Swiss
*aureliedellasanta@yahoo.com*
*www.aureliedellasanta.com*
Aurelie Dellasanta completed her undergraduate studies at HEAD, the Geneva University of Art and Design. She then moved to London to attend the Royal College of Art, appearing in the Show RCA 2011 and the accompanying catalogue and being highly commended in the Theo Fennell Awards. She has also exhibited extensively and won several grants throughout Switzerland. Recycling miscellaneous symbols and objects, Aurelie's engaging work critically scrutinizes behaviour and values that she sees as conflicting with the essence of humanity. > p. 111

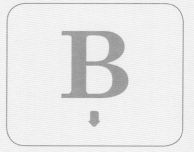

## BABETTE VON DOHNANYI
German
*info@bd-jewellery.com*
*www.bd-jewellery.eu*
Munich-born, Babette von Dohnanyi's career in jewelry-making began with diplomas in goldsmithing and casting under Bino Bini in Florence, where she later won First Prize at the 1997 International Handicrafts Trade Fair. She complemented this with an apprenticeship in silversmithing in Neugablonz, Germany and many seminars. Recent exhibition and book highlights include Lark Books' *500 Silver Jewelry Designs*. Babette's fascinating 'Polyp' series melds geometry and nature, establishing an interplay between robustness and flexibility in its allusions to polyp structures. > pp. 53, 163, 185, 206

## BARBARA AMZALLAG
Canadian
*bamzallag@gmail.com*
Born and educated in Montreal, Barbara Amzallag produces bold, sensual and refined work with multiple sources of inspiration. These include a personal legacy – her surname literally translates as 'makers of chains' – as well as historical awareness, a fixation with nature and architecture, and an annual pilgrimage to San Miguel de Allende, Mexico, whose vibrant creativity has significantly influenced her creations. Exploring the boundless possibilities offered by the interaction of metal and skin, she often spends several hours on a particular process as her pieces find their form.
> p. 108

## BARBARA CHRISTIE
Dutch
*blcjewel@aol.com*
*www.barbarachristie.com*
Utilizing precious metals and carefully sourced rare stones to fuse wearability and a sculpted look, Barbara Christie's one-of-a-kind pieces foreground movement, colour, tactility and their own creation process. A De Beers Diamond Competition winner, Barbara has even designed catwalk pieces for Tivoli and Valentino. A frequent exhibitor at London's Goldsmiths' Fair and SOFA New York, she is showcased in *The Earrings Book* and *Made to Wear* and has been teaching for over thirty years, including at Central Saint Martins and Morley College, both in London. > pp. 56, 61, 171

## BEATE KLOCKMANN
German
*beateklockmann@gmail.com*
*www.beateklockmann.com*
Beate Klockmann followed her goldsmithing training with jewelry-making studies at the Burg Giebichenstein University of Art and Design in Halle, Germany. Now a resident of Latour-de-France, she has had solo shows at the Marzee Gallery in the Netherlands, Caroline Van Hoek in Brussels and Ornamentum in Hudson, New York. Often labelled baroque, Beate's work embraces clear and chaotic forms, juxtaposing elements that are rarely combined. They embrace the pleasures of life, the beauty of the body and the landscape. > pp. 88, 93, 114, 164, 184

**BEATRIZ FABRES BARAHONA**
Chilean
*info@beatrizfabres.com*
*www.beatrizfabres.com*
Born in Santiago, Chile, Beatriz Fabres undertook
her jewelry education at the Le Arte Orafi School
in Florence, Italy. After completing her training,
she spent three years in Naples, a city with a rich
metalsmithing tradition, working both individually
and for other studios. In 2010 she embarked on a new
adventure in Spain, where she set up her own atelier.
Primarily worked in silver, combined with patina, dyed
horsehair or precious stones, her designs forge a sense
of harmony with the wearer's body. > pp. 44, 55, 106

**BEVERLY TADEU**
American
*bt@beverlytadeu.com*
*www.beverlytadeu.com*
New Jersey-born designer Beverly Tadeu is fascinated
by the myriad layers of meaning contained in the idea
of rootedness. At once sensual and down-to-earth,
her 'Rooted' collection consists of a range of gold and
oxidized silver pieces featuring intricate patterns and
interlaced threads, fusing durability and strength with
fragility and delicacy. Beverly has taken her work to
numerous exhibitions, including SOFA Chicago and
'In Line/In Metal' at New York's Aaron Faber Gallery
in 2011. She also appears in Lark Books' *500 Silver
Jewelry Designs.* > pp. 188, 189

**BIBA SCHUTZ**
American
*biba@bibaschutz.com | www.bibaschutz.com*
A design graduate from the American University in
Washington DC, Biba Schutz has garnered various
accolades during a career spanning more than
twenty-five years. A repeat exhibitor at SOFA, she
has showcased her work in several Lark Books titles,
in *Metalsmith* magazine and through solo shows at
the Gallery Loupe in New Jersey. Mixing precious
metals and handmade paper, Biba's recent work
delves into the beauty of imperfection. Using her
experiences and urban surroundings as a springboard,
her pieces enter into a dialogue with the viewer.
> pp. 42, 82, 103, 119, 121

**BLANCA SÁNCHEZ**
Spanish
*quieroestajoya@gmail.com*
*www.blancasanchez.com | www.peudereina.org*
Selected for the Françoise van den Bosch Foundation's
Young Talent Collection, Blanca Sánchez attended
the Madrid School of Art and Barcelona's Massana
School. She co-founded the Peu de Reina Contemporary
Jewelry Group, with which she has exhibited
collectively at home and abroad, and enjoyed her first
solo show at Barcelona's Alea Gallery in 2005. For
Blanca, the sine qua non of jewelry design is to spark
curiosity. To achieve this, she digs beneath the surface,
working against the grain and repurposing objects of
varied origin. > pp. 159, 206

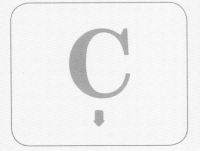

**CARACTÈRE** (Gema Barrera & Pascal Cretin)
Swiss
*info@galeriecaractere.com*
*www.galeriecaractere.com*
*www.madebycaractere.com*
Both graduates of a Higher School of Applied Arts
(in La Chaux-de-Fonds and Geneva respectively),
Gema Barrera and Pascal Cretin run Caractère, a
contemporary jewelry gallery in Neuchâtel with sales
outlets in three other locations across Switzerland.
Chalking up more than 55 exhibitions throughout
Europe and the US, they have also taught for over
ten years. Caractère's original pieces fuse innovation,
emotion and personal experiences. Classical music and
everyday items such as suction cups and water drops
have inspired some of their designs. > p. 165

**CARLES SERRANO – DELAJOIA**
Spanish
*carlesserrano@delajoia.com*
*www.delajoia.com*
Barcelona-born Carles Serrano studied in his hometown
at the Massana School and Industrial School, before
completing various workshops and opening his own
atelier. Carles is intrigued by the elaborate forms,
precision, symbolism and intricate workmanship of
classical jewelry. His designs aim to reflect the essence
of the past while putting a contemporary spin on it,
freeing it from superfluous ornamentation. He sees
jewelry-making as a way of forging one's own language,
creating an object that transforms the body while
eschewing superficiality. > pp. 65, 161

**CARMEN PINTOR**
Galeria Meko Joyería de Autor
Spanish
*info@galeriameko.com | www.galeriameko.com*
Born and educated in Santiago de Compostela, Carmen
Pintor subsequently moved to Barcelona, attending
the Llotja School and quickly establishing herself
on the local scene. She has contributed to wide-
ranging international exhibitions, including Velvet
da Vinci's 2004 touring show 'Anti-War Medals', and
to publications such as *New Rings*. Named a Master
Artisan by the Government of Catalonia in 2002,
she won the 2010 Catalan Federation of Jewelers,
Goldsmiths and Watchmakers' Artisan Award.
Carmen's meticulous designs draw heavily on the
colours, materials and textures of nature. > pp. 59, 167

**CAROLINA HORNAUER**
Chilean
*carohornauer@gmail.com*
Carolina studied architecture in her native Chile and
jewelry-making at Barcelona's Massana School. The
2008 SIERAAD New Traditional Jewellery contest
winner, Carolina participated in the 'Anti-War Medals'
show in New Orleans, Gray Area Jewelry's symposium
in Mexico City and the Society for Contemporary Crafts'
2011 exhibition 'Transformation 8: Contemporary
Works in Small Metals' in Pittsburgh. Fascinated
by handicrafts, details, and cabinets of curiosities,
Carolina often uses objects from flea markets and
family mementoes in her storytelling art jewelry. She
also alludes to Mapuche mythology and the earthquake
that decimated her home country in 2010. > pp. 10–11

**CATALINA BRENES**
Costa Rican
*catalina.brenes@gmail.com*
*www.catalinabrenes.com*
Qualified in both fine art and contemporary jewelry
design, Catalina Brenes unites European aesthetics –
mastered at Florence's Alchimia School – with Latin
American flair. Never losing sight of her roots, she
frequently recycles found materials, often combining
them with objects from her childhood. Her exhibition
credits include 'Collect' at London's Saatchi Gallery, the
two-person show 'Morfosi' at Barcelona's Alea Gallery
and the Bologna International Art Fair. Russia's *Free
Hugs* magazine dedicated six pages to her and she has
been spotlighted in several other publications. > p. 82

**CHRISTA LÜHTJE**
German
*c.luehtje@t-online.de*
*www.christaluehtje.de*
After apprenticing in Hamburg, her hometown, Christa
Lühtje studied at Munich's Academy of Fine Arts.
A career spanning over fifty years has been paved
with numerous awards, including the Bavarian State
Award, Hamburg's Edwin Scharff Prize and the City of
Munich's Cultural Promotion Prize, and exhibitions at
Jewelerswerk in Washington DC, and London's Saatchi
Gallery. Chiefly working with cut stones and gold, she
appears in Lark Books' *Masters: Gold* and her designs
aim to express the beauty of the world and capture
slices of life. > pp. 128, 184

**CHUN-LUNG HSIEH**
Taiwanese
*chunlung0513@gmail.com*
After graduating from Shu-Te University, Chun-
Lung Hsieh completed an MFA at Tainan National
University of the Arts. Playing with the way light and
colours reflect and refract on surfaces, his work so far
has amassed a range of distinctions, including a Silver
Award at the Asian Fashion Jewellery & Accessories
Design Competition, an honourable mention at the
2nd National Metal Crafts Competition and being
shortlisted for the 7th Cheongju International Craft
Biennale in Korea. He also features in Lark Books'
*500 Silver Jewelry Designs.* > p. 60

**COLLECTIVE FALABRAC**
Italian
*info@falabrac.it*
*www.falabrac.it*
Falabrac – Workshop of Ideas is a collective of young
designers who joined forces in 2010 to create quality
experimental jewelry. Their designs stem from a diverse
process in which members draw on their own expertise
and personal experience. Fusing traditional precious
metals and cutting-edge materials such as techno
nylon, their projects combine handcrafted techniques
with advanced technology such as 3D modelling and
rapid manufacturing methods. The group's work has
appeared in Spain's *Contemporary Jewellery Yearbook
2011* and at the 2011 JOYA fair in Barcelona. > p. 223

**CONSTANZA SOTO DONOSO**
Chilean
*constanzacl@gmail.com*
*constanzasotojoyas.blogspot.com*
Animal and cellular forms seep into the creative process
behind the work of Chilean designer Constanza Soto
Donoso, which represents a return to our underlying
origins. Since starting out at a local metalsmith's
atelier in 2009, Constanza has made intensive
progress. In 2010 she exhibited at Expoartesanía
Taller Sur, a regional crafts fair organized by the
Chilean government organization SERCOTEC, and in
2011 she took Second Place in the 2nd Copper Design
Contest, run by the Los Pelambres Mine and Santiago's
Contemporary Art Museum (MAC). > pp. 149, 156, 207

**CUCÚ RUIZ**
Spanish
*cucu@cucujoyas.com*
*www.cucujoyas.com*
A history of art graduate from the University of Seville,
Cucú Ruiz turned her attention to jewelry-making out
of artistic curiosity; it has now become her bona fide
passion. Aesthetic concerns shape her pieces, which
seek to engage the wearer in a creative communication
process, thereby forging bonds between object and user.
Having completed her professional jewelry training
at Florence's Le Arti Orafe school, Cucú has since
exhibited everywhere from Cyprus to East Yorkshire,
Milan and the prestigious Inhorgenta fair in Munich,
Germany. > pp. 144, 176

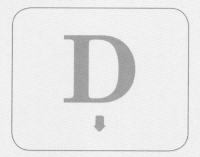

## DALILA GOMES
Portuguese
*dg.joiasdeautor@gmail.com*
The values of balance, versatility, precision and minimalism inform the work of Dalila Gomes, who is committed to exploring the process of making jewelry, rather than the end itself. Having studied for an undergraduate degree at the University of Oporto's Faculty of Architecture prior to pursuing training in jewelry design – her childhood passion – at the Contacto Directo School in Lisbon, Dalila uses a varied range of influences in her pieces, often blurring the lines between sculpture, architecture and painting. She is also heavily inspired by Japanese culture. > p. 90

.....................

## DAMIÀ MULET
Spanish
*damiamuletvanrell@hotmail.com*
Damià Mulet's designs are rooted in his native Balearic islands, highlighting the essence of the Mediterranean and often making use of local materials. He has won numerous prizes across Spain and the Balearic islands, earning First Prize at the 2005 and 2006 Palma de Mallorca Federation of Jewelry Makers and Watchmakers' Joya Mediterránea Competition and at Minorca's 2010 Es Mercadal Crafts Fair. He also boasts copious exhibition and teaching experience and currently heads the Art Jewelry Department at the School of Design of the Balearic Islands. > p. 54

.....................

## DANIEL DICAPRIO
American
*dandicaprio@gmail.com*
*www.dandicaprio.com*
Daniel DiCaprio is intrigued by unusual creatures and the way that organisms evolve within their environment, integrating these influences into his work. Combining precious metals with hardwoods, his pieces endeavour to make the viewer relate to the changes and transformations undergone during their creation. Daniel has been making jewelry since 2004, earning an MFA from East Carolina University in 2009 and exhibiting annually at SOFA together with Charon Kransen Arts since 2008. He has featured in Norwegian arts and crafts journal *Kunsthåndverk* and the prestigious *Metalsmith* magazine. > pp. 226, 227

.....................

## DAPHNE KRINOS
Greek
*daphnekrinos@aol.com*
*www.daphnekrinos.com*
Athens-born Daphne Krinos now lives and works in London and holds a degree from Middlesex University. City life (including architecture, urban structures, and street art) and memories of summers in Greece are the dual influences that inform her pieces, which seek to make the wearer feel unique. A regular exhibitor at the 'Collect' show, held at London's Saatchi Gallery and the Victoria & Albert Museum, Daphne has been featured in several Lark Books art jewelry titles. She gained a Gold Prize at the Goldsmiths' Company 2007 Craftsmanship and Design Awards. > pp. 60, 196, 197

## DENISE QUEIROZ
Brazilian
*denise@denisequeiroz.com*
*www.denisequeiroz.com*
After initially practising architecture, Denise Queiroz now designs jewelry for a living, graduating from SENAC (the National Commercial Apprenticeship Service) in Rio in 2008. These dual backgrounds, alongside multiple sources of inspiration including minimalism, organic forms, culture, nature, music and emotions, form the stimulus for her original concept pieces. Denise has contributed to several Brazilian publications and to exhibitions both at home – such as 2010's 'Joia Brasil' in Rio – and abroad, including the Brazilian jewelry showcase in late 2011 at the Brazilian Embassy in Berlin. > pp. 24, 145, 221

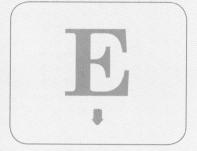

## EERO HINTSANEN
Finnish
*eero@chaoeero.com*
*www.chaoandeerojewel.com*
A goldsmithing graduate from the Institute of Design in Lahti, Finland, Eero Hintsanen produces meticulously crafted pieces that blend playfulness, seriousness and hints of urban style. He has been exhibiting since 1996, with recent highlights including 'The Plastic Show' at Velvet da Vinci, San Francisco, 'HIRAMEKI' at Tokyo's Living Design Center Ozone, and the 2009 show 'Finnish Jewellery 1600–2009' at the Design Museum, Helsinki. Major book credits include *500 Plastic Jewelry Designs* and *The Compendium Finale of Contemporary Jewellers*. > p. 116

.....................

## ELA BAUER
Polish
*ela@elabauer.com*
*www.elabauer.com*
Warsaw-born Ela Bauer moved to Amsterdam to attend the Gerrit Rietveld Academy. Forged in miscellaneous materials, with a recent penchant for silver, silicone and plastics, her designs probe the incompleteness of the world, highlighting the processes of development and disintegration at work around her. Besides taking her pieces to the likes of Schmuck in Munich, SOFA in the US and the European Prize for Applied Arts in Belgium, Ela has graced books including *Dreaming Jewellery* and Lark Books' *20th Century Jewelry: The Best of the 500 Series*. > p. 76

.....................

## ELISA PAIVA
Brazilian
*elisa_paiva@yahoo.com.br*
*www.elisapaiva.com*
After studying industrial design at the Federal University of Rio de Janeiro, Elisa Paiva moved on to courses in jewelry design and goldsmithing. 2009 was a breakthrough year for her, heralding appearances in the 'Design Contemporâneo Rio + França' exhibition, the 14th Craft Design fair in São Paulo and the book *Continuum: Design Contemporâneo no Rio de Janeiro*. Predominantly employing gold, silver and natural gemstones, Elisa casts her net wide for inspiration. She is constantly searching for innovative techniques to use on traditional materials. > pp. 43, 175

## ELVIRA LÓPEZ DEL PRADO
Spanish
*lopezdelprado@hotmail.com*
*www.lopezdelprado.com*
Following initial training in ceramics in Granada, Elvira López del Prado pursued a degree in public sculpture in Barcelona. The underlying strands of sculpture and ceramics, plus incursions into poetry, photography and painting, shape her exuberant, emotional and highly feminine pieces, which also often respond to geographical locations and small day-to-day occurrences. Now a resident of Flagstaff, Arizona, Elvira has exhibited extensively and is the author of two books in Spanish publishing house Parramón's *Decorative Techniques* series, on costume jewelry and felt. > p. 191

.....................

## EMILY WATSON
American
*mail1@metalemily.com*
*www.metalemily.com*
Influenced by anatomy and geography, Emily Watson's hand-hewn pieces are considered and tactile, moulding themselves to the wearer's body. She often combines conventional and innovative materials, frequently harnessing industrial cast-offs in order to turn them into something precious. An MFA holder from the State University of New York, New Paltz, Emily has shown her work at events including Craftboston and the American Craft Council Show. *New Rings*, *500 Enameled Objects* and *500 Plastic Jewelry Designs* are among her book credits. > pp. 66, 99, 173, 215

.....................

## ENRIC MAJORAL
Spanish
*www.majoral.com*
A recipient of the 2007 Spanish National Crafts Award and the title of Master Artisan from the Government of Catalonia, Enric Majoral is one of the most highly regarded designers in Spain. His pieces have been exhibited worldwide and have been acquired by the permanent collection at New York's Museum of Arts and Design (MAD). Working from his atelier-cum-showroom on the island of Formentera, Enric utilizes essential lines to forge sensual, elegant, often unique designs that ally his personal world view with Mediterranean flair. > pp. 123, 159, 185, 201, 217

.....................

## ESTELA GUITART
Spanish
*estela.guitart@gmail.com*
*estelaguitart.com*
Barcelona-born Estela Guitart made her first forays into jewelry design from 1988–90 after obtaining a grant to attend Milan's Istituto Europeo di Design. After returning home, she completed numerous courses at the Massana School, and served for several years on the board of the distinguished Orfebres FAD contemporary jewelry association. Her 'Just Married' wedding rings earned an honourable mention at the 24th Expohogar in 2004. Merging function, creativity and repetition, Estela seeks to unlock the full potential of the jewelry she produces. > p. 155

.....................

## ESTER FAIMAN
Estonian
*ester@rada7.ee*
Ester Faiman trained for a BA in Jewellery and Blacksmithing and an MFA in Interdisciplinary Arts at the Estonian Academy of Arts, with a sojourn at Edinburgh College of Art sandwiched between these experiences. Featured in *The Compendium Finale of Contemporary Jewellers*, she has participated in numerous group and solo exhibitions, including a recent one-woman show at Tallinn's A-Galerii. Broaching issues such as conflicts of identity, Esther's work deploys varied techniques, often drawing inspiration from photography, video, sculpture, land art and site-specific installations. > pp. 92, 100

## EVA BURTON
Argentinian
*evaburtonjoyas@gmail.com*
*www.evaburtonjoyas.com.ar*
*evaburtonjoyasdeautor.blogspot.com*
Buenos Aires native Eva Burton boasts an impressively varied portfolio of training, culminating in studies at Barcelona's Massana School. This includes courses in modern, contemporary and art jewelry and classes in techniques such as lost-wax casting, acid etching, chiselling and art restoration and materials including amber, resins, porcelain and enamel. Committed to venturing into the unknown, Eva has a love of experimentation that drives her highly personal work, in which she views the wearer as the recipient of a message containing a piece of herself. > p. 74

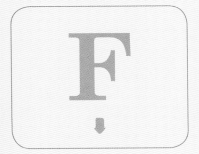

## FANNY AGNIER
French
*fannyagnier@gmail.com*
*www.fannyagnier.com*
A graduate of Geneva University of Art and Design, Fanny Agnier began making jewelry in 2005. Having apprenticed under Philip Sajet and learned granulation under Giovanni Corvaja, she is currently turning her attention to new techniques and materials in her pursuit of perfection. Putting a contemporary spin on classical techniques, Fanny's designs are largely worked in gold, silver and enamel. She has showcased her work at Amsterdam's Galerie Louise Smit, at the Gallery of Art in Legnica, Poland and at the Gallery Deux Poissons in Tokyo. > pp. 80, 88, 110

## FEDERICO CASTRILLÓN
Colombian
*federico.castrillon@gmail.com*
*www.vivalalibertad.com*
Federico Castrillón studied advertising at the Pontifical Bolivarian University in Medellín, his hometown. He currently splits his time between his jewelry brand, La Libertad, founded in 2006, and freelance graphic design. The annual collections that Federico produces for La Libertad intermingle vintage Baroque and Renaissance ornamentation with more modern influences such as Art Deco and Art Nouveau. His designs often take inspiration from the natural world; examples include the 'Ornithology' and 'Savage Carnivorism' collections, which explore the roles played by animals in different human cultures. > pp. 16, 17

## FELIEKE VAN DER LEEST
Dutch
*felieke@feliekevanderleest.com*
*www.feliekevanderleest.com*
Juxtaposing precious metals and plastics with textile techniques, Felieke van der Leest has forged her own idiom over the last fifteen years. Now living and working in Øystese, Norway, she draws on the memory of childhood visits to the zoo in the Netherlands, her metalsmithing training in Schoonhoven and her studies at Amsterdam's Gerrit Rietveld Academy, where she unleashed her imagination. A veteran of numerous exhibitions, Felieke creates collector's pieces that can be purchased at galleries in New York, Tokyo and Amsterdam. > p. 72

## FERRAN IGLESIAS
Spanish
*atelieriglesias@telefonica.net*
*www.atelierferraniglesias.com*
Born in Terrassa, near Barcelona, Ferran Iglesias made his first moves in the world of jewelry design with a goldsmithing apprenticeship in Santiago de Chile, building on this experience with studies at Barcelona's Massana School and Llotja School. His intricately crafted pieces are inspired by the rhythmic elements that recur in nature. A finalist at Inhorgenta 2011, in Munich, Ferran has graced various international exhibitions and fairs, including recently in Neuwied and Stipshausen, both in Germany, as well as several specialist magazines and books. > pp. 20, 22, 23

## FRANCE ROY
Canadian
*fr-roy@videotron.ca*
Montreal Jewellery School graduate France Roy probes beneath the surface of existence to make work that is relevant to contemporary life. Her distinctive pieces habitually combine found objects and coloured epoxy resins with precious metals. France has picked up multiple distinctions throughout her career, including a nomination for the Prix du Québec lifetime achievement award in 2011 and an honourable mention at Toronto's Northern Lights Exhibition. Featured in the 2011 volume *New Rings*, she held a major solo show in 2008 at Montreal's Noel Guyomarc'h Gallery. > pp. 170, 177

## FRÉDÉRIQUE COOMANS
Belgian
*info@frederiquecoomans.com*
*www.frederiquecoomans.com*
Up-and-coming Brussels-born creator Frédérique Coomans studied fashion design at Francisco Ferrer High School and contemporary jewelry at the Brussels Institute of Arts and Crafts. Awarded the 2009 Tremplin Prize for recent Belgian art school graduates, she was featured in France's 'Jeunes Talents du Nord' exhibition and EUNIQUE in Karlsruhe, Germany in 2010. Aiming to plunge viewers into a new dimension, Frédérique interweaves the dual strands of her training in her playful work. A regular exponent of upcycling, she also incorporates dashes of surrealism. > pp. 87, 203

## GABRIELA BARRÓN OLVERA
Mexican
*gabybojoyas@hotmail.com*
After studying industrial design at the Ibero-American University, in her hometown of Torreón – winning the Mexican Government's Nazario Ortiz Garza Medal for Academic Excellence – Gabriela Barrón Olvera turned to jewelry-making. This vocation is firmly bound up with the history of her family, four generations of whom mined silver and minerals. Digging into the essence of the Mexican desert, Gabriela harnesses properties such as light, purity, warmth, simplicity, elusiveness and defiance as the keynotes of her attempt to engage viewers intimately with this landscape. > p. 156

## GERALDINE NISHI
Canadian
*gerinishi@yahoo.com*
*www.geraldinenishi.com*
Holder of a BFA in Painting and Sculpture from Canada's University of Victoria, Geraldine Nishi studied jewelry design in Florence at the prestigious Alchimia School, winning the school's Alchimia Quaternitas Prize for her work at the Galerie Sofie Lachaert in Ghent, Belgium, where she exhibited solo. She was present at Schmuck 2011 in Munich, Germany, and featured in the June 2011 edition of *Mercedes-Benz Magazine Thailand*. Geraldine's work is a celebration of feasts or, to be more precise, the joy and spectacle of growing, cooking and eating food. > p. 103

## GERTI MACHACEK
Austrian
*gerti.machacek@atelier-machacek.at*
*www.atelier-machacek.at*
After majoring in history of art at the University of Vienna, Gerti Machacek launched into jewelry design with a goldsmithing apprenticeship under Hans Muliar. With over twenty-five years' exhibition experience, her career highlights include the 1992 Austrian State Prize for Crafts and appearances in books such as *Art Meets Jewellery* and *Schmuck: Kunst am Körper*. Imbuing her pieces with movement and portability, Gerti produces highly sculptural work that interacts with the body and serves as a mark of identity or a memento. > pp. 173, 219

## GILLIAN E. BATCHER
Canadian
*gillian@pash.ca*
*www.pash.ca | pashjewellery.blogspot.com*
As well as boasting a degree in psychology from the University of Western Ontario, multi-award-winning designer Gillian E. Batcher graduated with distinction from the Jewellery Arts Program at George Brown College, Toronto. On graduating, she spent three years as an artist in residence at Toronto's Harbourfront Centre, and she has exhibited widely across the US and Canada. She now combines making jewelry under the PASH Jewellery Design brand with teaching goldsmithing at her studio, OCAD University and George Brown College. > p. 157

## GUNTIS LAUDERS
Latvian
*gallery@putti.lv*
*www.lauders.lv*
*www.puti.lv*
Masterfully mixing silver with materials including coral, mammoth ivory, ebony and assorted stones, Guntis Lauders's jewelry teems with symbolic associations, stemming from his absorption of different cultures during his formative years in Latvia and Estonia. Riga-born, Guntis has exhibited both solo – at Riga's Putti Gallery – and as part of a group in locations including Madrid. He has amassed several prizes, including notably First Prize at the 1991 Tallinn Applied Art Triennial and Riga City Council's Jewelry Designer of the Year Award in 1998. > p. 36

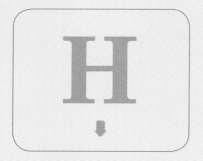

## HELLA GANOR
Israeli
*hella@hellaganor.com*
*www.hellaganor.com*
A French language and literature graduate from Tel Aviv University, Hella Ganor switched her focus to jewelry design in 1986, winning a national competition the following year. She is now based in Herzliya, but many of her career milestones have come in New York and Tel Aviv – in the latter she has held several exhibitions, including a solo sculpture show, launched the Netline series in 2011 and run the L'ORO gallery and showroom. Hella's sensual, elaborate work explores the overlap between sculpture and jewelry, adorning and interacting with the body. > p. 48

## HUI-MEI PAN
Taiwanese
*panhm@yahoo.com*
*www.panstyle.com*
Born in Tainan, Taiwan, Hui-Mei Pan holds an MFA in Metals and Jewelry Design from the Savannah College of Art and Design in Georgia, USA. She draws heavily on her culture and background in her elaborate, organic designs, which she has showcased in the US, the UK and Hong Kong, in *New Rings* and in two volumes from Lark Books' *500* series. Beyond jewelry-making, Hui-Mei Pan has published and illustrated award-winning children's books, including *Piggy in My Pocket* and *What's in Grandma's Grocery Bag?* > pp. 14, 121

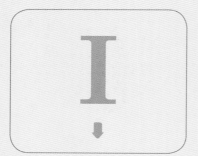

## IMMA GIBERT
Spanish
*imma@immagibert.com*
*www.immagibert.com*
Designer and educator Imma Gibert studied at Barcelona's Massana School and the University of Barcelona, opening her own studio-cum-workshop in 1980. In 2002 she travelled to Denver to exhibit her work and attend a fold-forming workshop with Charles Lewton-Brain. She has contributed to several books, including *New Rings*, and to major shows in Japan and Spain. Imma avidly sketches her ideas before producing her creations, which ally strength and expressiveness. Her pieces have evolved from a symbolic, allegorical aesthetic to a more personal style. > p. 40

## IÑAKI SALOM
Spanish
*info@inakisalom.com*
*www.inakisalom.com*
After studying fine art at the University of Barcelona, Iñaki Salom obtained a Master's in Graphic Design and took up jewelry-making at the Catalan Federation of Jewelers, Goldsmiths and Watchmakers. He founded his own jewelry atelier/showroom in Barcelona in 2007, in the wake of previous experiences as an art teacher and graphic designer. Iñaki is fascinated by typography, which he imports into the world of jewelry through a process in which letters are turned into sculptures and moulded in myriad materials. > p. 204

## IRIS SAAR ISAACS
Israeli
*iris@insyncdesign.com.au*
*www.insyncdesign.com.au*
Tel Aviv native Iris Saar Isaacs lives and trained in Melbourne, Australia, receiving the Melbourne Design Award in 2010 and featuring in books such as *Handmade in Melbourne* and *The Melbourne Design Guide*. She has exhibited extensively both within Australia and abroad, including in Frankfurt and Milan. The 2010 Faces of Design Award (Berlin) and a place in Spain's *Contemporary Jewellery Yearbook 2011* are two other recent highlights. Harnessing natural beauty, organic forms and asymmetry, Iris's work expresses the contrast between inner and outer worlds. > p. 83

## IRO KASKANI
Cypriot
*iro.kaskani@cytanet.com.cy*
*www.irokaskani.com*
Broaching ideas related to space, lack of symmetry and scale, Iro Kaskani's interstitial pieces marry precious and non-precious materials in their quest to forge intimate physical links with the human body. Iro completed an MA in Architecture before undertaking a course in jewelry design in Florence, Italy. She now runs her own workshop/gallery in her hometown of Nicosia, as well as exhibiting at fairs in Cyprus, Germany (Inhorgenta, Munich), Italy and Denmark (Brand New Copenhagen). She features in Lark Books' *500 Plastic Jewelry Designs*. > pp. 144, 215

## ISA DUARTE RIBEIRO
Portuguese
*lab.d.arte@gmail.com*
A multi-award-winner educated at Lisbon University, Isa Duarte Ribeiro combines jewelry-making with painting, lecturing and writing for art magazines. She has appeared in multiple exhibitions and books such as *New Rings* and *As esperanças plásticas portuguesas*. Isa's pieces have been acquired by a range of museums and art venues, including notably Lisbon's National Museum of Costume and Fashion and its Design and Fashion Museum (MUDE). Her recent work, encompassing jewelry, drawings and installations, has been inspired by surrealist philosopher and writer Georges Bataille. > p. 95

## ISABELLE FUSTINONI
French
*isafusti@hotmail.fr*
A passionate observer, Isabelle Fustinoni seeks to discover what lies beneath the surface of everyday scenes. Another of her passions is Africa, where she lived and picked up numerous local jewelry-making techniques. All of these influences come to bear on her work, which focuses on the contrasts, complementarities, properties and flaws of different techniques and raw materials. Born in Longwy, France, Isabelle studied at the School of Decorative Arts in Strasbourg, where she is now based. > p. 67

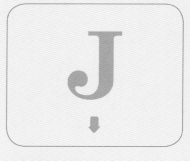

## J. ADRIANNE DIENNO
American
*adienno@gmail.com*
*www.jadriannedienno.com*
With a particular penchant for the use of married metals, including nickel, silver, gold, brass and copper, J. Adrianne Dienno attempts to channel the beauty she perceives around her into her pieces, as well as drawing stimulation from her Indian cultural background. She trained and began making jewelry at Northern Arizona University in 2008, subsequently showcasing her work in the 2010 exhibition 'Winter Wonders', at San Diego's Taboo Gallery, and in 2011 at the Artists' Gallery in Flagstaff, Arizona. > pp. 52, 171

## JACKIE ANDERSON
Canadian
*juell1@shaw.ca*
Jackie Anderson studied in her hometown of Calgary, Canada, attending the Alberta College of Art and Design (ACAD), who later gave her an Alumni Award of Excellence. Colours, culture, cityscapes, structures, stories and personal passions provide the creative spark for her acclaimed work. Jackie has taught, mentored, lectured and exhibited widely, including the solo eyewear show 'Making a Spectacle of Myself' as well as award-winning contributions to the jewelry exhibitions 'Inspired By' and the Metal Arts Guild of Canada's 'MAG 2067 – Crafting the Future'. > pp. 48, 107

## JACQUELINE I. LILLIE
Austrian
*plillie@hotmail.com*
A graduate of Vienna's Academy of Applied Arts, Jacqueline I. Lillie has seen her work grace museums worldwide and books including *The History of Beads* and *The New Beadwork*. She has twice been honoured by *Ornament* magazine, and has also completed award-winning commissions for Sydney's Powerhouse Museum and New York's Corning Museum of Glass. Combining small antique glass beads and precision-engineered metal components, Jacqueline's pieces fuse art, industry, function, flexibility and personality. She counts Bauhaus, the Soviet Constructivists, the textiles of Mali and the Wiener Werkstätte among her influences. > pp. 24, 151, 205

## JAN SMITH
Canadian
*jansmithca@hotmail.com* | *www.jansmith.ca*
Canadian enamel specialist Jan Smith espouses the notion of art jewelry as public art that engages viewers in an exchange involving colour, movement, touch and sound. Jan was educated at Penland School of Crafts, North Carolina and at NSCAD University in Halifax, Canada. Honoured at the Northern California Enamel Guild International Juried Enamel Exhibition (twice) and the 9th Biennial International Juried Enamel Exhibition, her work has graced numerous top jewelry forums, from SOFA Chicago to Velvet da Vinci, San Francisco, and two Lark Books titles. > pp. 171, 195

## JANIS VILKS
Latvian
*gallery@putti.lv*
*www.putti.lv*
Combining precious metals, natural stones and miscellaneous gem-cutting and setting techniques, Janis Vilks is open to users and viewers taking away their own meanings from his pieces. Janis commenced his studies at the Art Academy of Latvia, before specializing in metal design at the Riga School of Design and Art. Regularly exhibiting at Riga's Putti Gallery, he has also displayed his work at the Latvian Embassy in Oslo, Norway. He won the Grand Prix at the 1999 Prague Quadrennial of Performance Design and Space. > p. 37

## JAROSLAV KUČERA
Czech
*jaroslavkucera@hotmail.com*
*www.kow.cz | www.envelopebijoux.com*
Jaroslav Kučera's jewelry-making career goes back to when he began studying at the Secondary School of Applied Arts in Turnov, at the age of fourteen. He then progressed to the University of Applied Arts in Prague, before heading to the US to study metal design at Miami University, Ohio. Jaroslav channels the power of particular materials and simple forms in order to fashion unexpected and compellingly beautiful designs. These have been exhibited in his native Prague, in Miami and at the likes of the Silver Triennial in Hanau, Germany. > p. 91

## JENNACA DAVIES
American
*contact@jennaca.com*
*www.jennaca.com*
Though mainly focused on jewelry-making, Rhode Island School of Design graduate Jennaca Davies has multiple strings to her bow. In 2007 the American Austrian Foundation awarded her a scholarship to attend the Salzburg International Summer Academy, and she spent a semester in 2008 as artist-in-residence at the Oregon College of Art (OCAC), practising electroforming and designing a small jewelry range. Also a part-time architect, she holds Bachelors of Architecture and Building Sciences from New York's Rensselaer Polytechnic Institute. > pp. 94, 205

## JESSE BERT
American
*jessedanielbert@gmail.com*
*www.jessebert.com*
Jesse Bert earned a BFA and MFA in Metals Design from the Rochester Institute of Technology and East Carolina University respectively, before moving to Mexico. Frequently utilizing found and repurposed objects, his highly sculptural jewelry is largely inspired by his natural surroundings – indeed, when not teaching or designing, he is passionate about exploring the Mexican countryside and mountains. Interviewed in the Mexican magazine *JOYA* in June 2011, Jesse has participated in numerous exhibitions in Mexico, as well as the 2011 Silver Festival in Legnica, Poland. > pp. 213, 220

## JOANNE HAYWOOD
British
*joannehaywood51@hotmail.com*
*www.joannehaywood.co.uk*
*theneedlefiles.blogspot.com*
The author of *Mixed Media Jewellery*, Joanne Haywood is renowned for her designs that interweave textiles and metals. A contributor to many exhibitions and books, she trained at London's Central Saint Martins and also has a Postgraduate Certificate in Education from Greenwich University. Captivated by the way humans interact with objects as well as rituals, identity, memories and transformation, Joanne uses contrasting and contradictory forms to explore the essence of materials and ideas of permanence. > pp. 99, 132, 133

## JOHN BLAIR
Canadian
*jblairdesign@shaw.ca*
John Blair built on his education at Alberta College of Art and Design in Calgary, Canada – who subsequently granted him an Alumni Award of Excellence in 2002 – by attending San Francisco's Revere Academy of Jewelry Arts. He has been featured in books including *500 Metal Vessels* and exhibitions from Toronto to Calgary and Washington DC. A purveyor of elaborate, timeless designs, in 2005 he was commissioned to make the ceremonial knife that Queen Elizabeth II used to cut a cake marking the province of Alberta's centenary celebrations. > p. 49

## JORGE MANILLA
Mexican
*manillajorge@yahoo.com*
*www.jorgemanilla.com*
Incorporating porcelain, silver, paper and dried cactus, Jorge Manilla's creations are a syncretic combination of Catholicism and Aztec culture, blurring the lines between jewelry and objects. Issues such as attraction, repulsion, fear, life and death coalesce in his work. Jorge studied classical jewelry in Mexico, before relocating to Belgium to continue his training. Currently a teacher at the Royal Academy of Fine Arts in Antwerp and Rhok Academy in Brussels, he has held countless exhibitions worldwide. In 2010 he won the prestigious Henry Van de Velde Award. > p. 120

## JOSÉE DESJARDINS
Canadian
*jd.bijoux@hotmail.com*
Canada-based Josée Desjardins imbues her distinctive designs with personal experiences (whether lived or imagined) and intimate connections with organic and social life. A major recent collection and exhibition, 'A Jeweller's Travel Memorabilia', bears out this trend. A graduate from Montreal Art Jewelry and Metalsmithing School (EJMAM), Josée is currently pursuing a Master's in Psychosocial Practices at the University of Quebec in Rimouski (UQAR). Book credits include *New Rings*, *The Best of the 500 Series* and *Ornament and Object: Canadian Jewellery and Metal Art 1946–1996*. > p. 75

## JOSEP RAVENTÓS
Spanish
*learagroup@gmail.com*
*josepraventos.blogspot.com*
Josep Raventós has completed many courses dedicated to specific materials and processes such as electroplating, chiselling, high-temperature furnace construction and gemmology at schools in his native Barcelona, including the Llotja School and the Autonomous University. He is certified by the Federation of European Education in Gemmology. A firm believer that there is a right material for each piece, Josep derives great satisfaction from projecting his unconscious thoughts and experiences into his work, which also takes its lead from nature, music and poetry. > p. 166

## JUDY McCAIG
British
*judymccaig@gmail.com*
Joint recipient of the First Prize at the 19th International Jewellery Competition in Legnica, Poland, Edinburgh-born designer Judy McCaig produces mixed-media designs inspired by her travels and her reactions to natural phenomena. Now a resident of Barcelona, Judy studied in Dundee, Scotland, before completing an MA at the Royal College of Art in London. As well as attending Schmuck in Munich, her recent milestones include taking part in the exhibition 'Castelli, miniature, astri ed alchimia' in Padua, for which she also featured in the catalogue, and the books *500 Pendants* and *New Rings*. > p. 169

## JÚLIA COMPTE
Spanish
*juliacomptepamies@gmail.com*
*www.juliacomptejoies.com*
*juliacomptejoies.blogspot.com*
Júlia Compte fashions simple and precise pieces imbued with the spirit of contemporary designers and influenced by geometric forms, nature and Op Art. Júlia learned her trade at the School of Art and Design in Tarragona, in her native Catalonia. She is a repeat exhibitor at Inhorgenta, Munich (2006–2009) and EuroBijoux, Minorca, and has also been showcased at the JOYA Barcelona Contemporary Jewelry Week. Her work has been published in the book *New Rings* and in *Casa Viva* magazine. > p. 148

## JULIA DEVILLE
New Zealander
*julia@discemori.com | www.discemori.com*
New Zealand-born, Julia deVille holds an Advanced Diploma in Gold and Silversmithing from NMIT, Melbourne, and a qualification from the Gemmological Association of Australia. Her work graces the books *Handmade in Melbourne*, *New Directions in Jewellery II* and *Bijoux, illustration et design*, and has been exhibited throughout Australia. Fascinated by memento mori and Victorian death adornments, Julia combines classical materials with elements that were once alive. Stressing her focus on preserving beauty, for her taxidermy she exclusively uses animals that have died of natural causes. > pp. 34, 77, 182, 193

## JULIANA ESTRADA LONDOÑO
Colombian
*fenn@une.net.co*
*www.fenn.com.co*
Nature is the driving force behind the work of Colombian designer Juliana Estrada Londoño, who loves to unveil the hidden charm within her natural sources of inspiration. Her exotic, one-of-a-kind pieces utilize a varied range of colours, patterns and materials – from silver to resins, fruit seeds and semi-precious stones – so that every wearer can make her designs their own. Juliana trained in jewelry-making and industrial design at schools including the Bolivarian Pontifical University in her native Medellín. She spent one semester in Europe as part of her studies. > p. 158

## JUN HU
Chinese
*wawajun1212@yahoo.com.cn*
*www.gameofmetal.com*
Chiefly, though not exclusively, inspired by nature, Jun Hu's pieces seek to keep alive threatened elements of Chinese culture while wedding them to modern urban and Western trends. To do so, he harnesses the likes of wood, natural stones, resin and many other materials alongside precious metals. Jun is a Beijing Institute of Fashion Technology MA graduate with numerous major international exhibitions under his belt, including several top fairs in Beijing. Book credits include *New Rings*, *500 Earrings* and *500 Plastic Jewelry Designs*. > pp. 111, 151

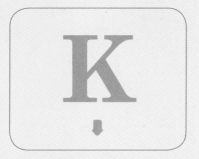
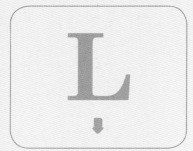

## KARIM OUKID OUKSEL
Algerian
*arteyani@gmail.com*
*www.karimoukid.com*
Boasting a free, independent style, born out of his use of geometric patterns worked in traditional filigree style, Algeria-born Karim Oukid Ouksel's work is intimately linked with his homeland and culture. Karim studied in Tizi Ouzou, in his mother country, before moving to Barcelona, where he taught Kabyle Berber jewelry-making at the Massana School. He has exhibited across Europe, Algeria and the US, and is showcased in the 2011 *Santa Fe International Folk Art Market Magazine* and in Carles Codina's book *Aula de joyería*.
> p. 51

## KARIN SEUFERT
German
*kgseufert@gmx.de | www.karinseufert.de*
Karin Seufert's jewelry aims to reappropriate commoditized images, blurring the lines between the recognizable and the unrecognizable and altering ways of seeing. Karin was educated in the Netherlands, first in Schoonhoven and later at Amsterdam's Gerrit Rietveld Academy. A contributor to the books *New Directions in Jewellery II*, numerous Lark Books volumes, *Bijoux, illustration et design* and *New Rings*, she has been exhibiting her work for over twenty-five years in places including Tokyo, Seoul and throughout her native Germany. She has also been honoured by Frankfurt's International Jewellery Competition and Poland's Legnica Gallery of Art. > pp. 96, 115

## KATJA PRINS
Dutch
*www.katjaprins.com*
Katja Prins's work probes the considerable overlap between bodies and machines, the corporeal and the mechanical, as technology and industry are increasingly utilized to improve the body. A graduate from the Vakschool in Schoonhoven and Amsterdam's Gerrit Rietveld Academy, Katja has exhibited solo both at home – in Leiden and Amsterdam – and at the Ornamentum gallery in Hudson, New York. Major publication credits include a 128-page monograph, *The Uncanny Valley*, published by Darling Publications, who named her its Jeweller of the Year in 2009.
> p. 216

## KVETOSLAVA FLORA SEKANOVA
Slovakian
*kvietok50@gmail.com*
*kvetoslava-flora-sekanova.weebly.com*
Regularly utilizing recycled newsprint and processes such as hollowing, carving, surface manipulation and reconstruction, Kvetoslava Flora Sekanova's work provides poetic solutions to bridge the gap between jewelry and everyday phenomena. Her pieces are mysterious, personal and very wearable. Slovakia-born, Kvetoslava lived in the US, the UK and Australia before settling in New Zealand, winning several awards at the Hungry Creek School of Art, near Auckland. She was selected for Talente 2010 in Munich and placed second at the 2011 Objective Art Awards. > p. 122

## L. SUE SZABO
American
*lsueszabo@hotmail.com*
*www.lsueszabo.com*
L. Sue Szabo studied metalsmithing at the Museum of Art in Toledo, Ohio, where she is now based. Featured in Lark Books' *500 Necklaces* and *500 Gemstone Jewels*, she won two awards from *Lapidary Journal Jewelry Artist* magazine in 2010, while major showcases include the Biennial International Juried Enamel Exhibition and the Annual Contemporary Crafts Exhibition in Mesa, Arizona. No potential influence is lost on her and she prizes experimentation in her colourful, eclectic and frequently playful work, which boldly reinterprets essentially simple forms. > pp. 215, 220

## LARITZA GARCIA
American
*littlefairblue@gmail.com*
The interaction between colour and the urban backdrop – notably the graffiti, neon, murals and handpainted signs that permeate her landscape – inform Laritza Garcia's recent body of work, which engages in a form of layered cultural dialogue punctuated by vivid, luminescent tones expressed chiefly through powder-coated copper and sterling silver. Laritza earned a BFA in Metal Design from Texas State University, before moving to Greenville, North Carolina, to embark on postgraduate studies at East Carolina University.
> p. 119

## LAURA EYLES
Australian
*lauraeyles@hotmail.com*
*lauraeyles.blogspot.com*
Taking her lead from mechanical engineering, Laura Eyles creates work that is ingenious and functional, regaling the viewer and wearer with clever mechanics that always contain a hidden reward to serve as a counterpart to the beautiful materials employed. Laura studied painting, gold and silversmithing and jewelry engineering in Melbourne at RMIT University and the Northern Melbourne Institute of TAFE (NMIT). Her exhibition highlights so far are the NMIT Graduate Exhibition in 2010 and 'Contemporary Australian Silver & Metalwork', the 11th Biennial Ernest Leviny Commemorative Silver Exhibition. > pp. 115, 145

## LEONOR HIPÓLITO
Portuguese
*contact@leonorhipolito.com*
*www.leonorhipolito.com*
Lisbon native Leonor Hipólito combines jewelry-making with lecturing and teaching both at home, in cities such as Lisbon and Oporto, and abroad. She learned jewelry design at Amsterdam's Gerrit Rietveld Academy, obtaining the Gerrit Rietveld Award, and has also spent time at New York's Parsons The New School of Design and the University of Applied Sciences in Trier, Germany. Juxtaposing expression and introspection, Leonor conceives jewelry as a bridge between the world and the self, and as a vehicle for emotions and ideas.
> pp. 89, 154, 173

## LIAUNG-CHUNG YEN
Taiwanese
*liaung@yahoo.com | www.liaungchungyen.com*
Taiwan-born Liaung-Chung Yen eschews concrete meanings in favour of heavily sculptural jewelry that interweaves beauty, stillness and illumination. Holding an MFA in Metal and Jewelry from the Savannah College of Art and Design in Georgia, Liaung-Chung is a two-time NICHE Awards finalist and was awarded a New York Foundation for the Arts Fellowship in 2005. He has contributed to eight titles in Lark Books' *500* series and his work has been showcased at SOFA Chicago and West, the German Recycling Design Prize and Oslo, Norway's National Museum of Art, Architecture and Design. > pp. 20, 163, 221

## LIESBET BUSSCHE
Belgian
*info@liesbetbussche.com*
*www.liesbetbussche.com*
The dual cues for Liesbet Bussche's designs are reflections on jewelry itself – namely its context, history, value and its relationship with its wearer – and the city as a stage for the exploration of public and private boundaries. Born in Antwerp, Liesbet graduated from Amsterdam's Gerrit Rietveld Academy. As well as exhibiting throughout her native Belgium and in the Netherlands, the US, Nepal, Taiwan and Sweden, she has contributed to the books *Urban Interventions: Personal Projects in Public Spaces* and *Belgium is Design: Design for Mankind*. > p. 125

## LIISA HASHIMOTO
American
*hinge@sage.ocn.ne.jp*
*www.hinge-dept.com*
A native of Austin, Texas, Liisa Hashimoto graduated from the School of the Museum of Fine Arts in Boston. She now lives in Osaka, Japan, where she holds an annual solo showcase at the Espace 446. Other major credits include a solo show at e.g.etal in Melbourne, Australia, the book *Dreaming Jewelry* and an international conceptual jewelry exhibition at the Putti Gallery in Riga, Latvia. Her predominantly nature-inspired pieces have twice earned awards at Japan's Itami International Craft Exhibition.
> pp. 121, 176

## LILI ZSABOKORSZKY
Hungarian
*zsabokorszkylili@gmail.com*
Based on pure forms, Lila Zsabokorszky's work explores the functionality and wearability of jewelry through the varied rhythms of different materials and shapes. Lili was educated at the Vocational Training School and the Metal Design Faculty of the Moholy-Nagy University of Art and Design, both in her hometown of Budapest. Her career landmark achievements have chiefly come in the city, including several prize-winning contest entries and exhibitions at the Sterling and Ponton Galleries, among others. > pp. 71, 202

## LINNÉA ERIKSSON
Swedish
*info@linneaeriksson.se*
*www.linneaeriksson.se*
Linnéa Eriksson obtained a BA in Jewelry Art at the School of Design and Crafts in Gothenburg, Sweden. During her studies she won several grants, including one from the Estrid-Ericson Foundation (2010) to spend a semester at Rhode Island School of Design in the US. Featured in publications such as *500 Silver Jewelry Designs*, Linnéa's pieces are responses to stimuli in her surroundings, from dashes of colour to scraps of metal and urban surfaces. She aims to leave her footprint behind for posterity.
> pp. 97, 187

## LISA BLACK
American
*lisa@lisablackjewellery.com*
*www.lisablackjewellery.com*
A passion for antiquities and a commitment to ornament underpin the pursuits of New York-born Lisa Black, now resident in Byron Bay, Australia. She frequently restores rare items from bygone eras, including turquoise melon and Egyptian faience beads, South Sea Keshi pearls, and chalcedony. Boasting diverse training in fine art, architecture, jewelry and horticulture, Lisa Black has exhibited at New York's Aaron Faber Gallery and Museum of Arts and Design (MAD) and Sydney's Annandale Galleries. Publication credits include *The Robb Report* and *The Australian Financial Review.* > pp. 28, 39, 42, 57, 67

## LISA M. JOHNSON
American
*lisamjohnsonart@gmail.com*
*www.lisamjohnsonart.com*
*arrowmontresidents.blogspot.com*
Combining metalsmithing and ceramic techniques, Lisa M. Johnson frequently attempts to redefine the recognizable by reworking common objects. Her pieces are stimulating, alluring and sometimes humorous. Lisa obtained a BFA and MFA in Metals and Jewelry Design at Miami University and Indiana University respectively. She has completed several artistic residencies, has exhibited domestically and abroad (Riga, Latvia) and is featured in the books *Plastic Jewelry, Silver Jewelry* and *Humor in Craft.* > p. 93

## LLUÍS DURAN
Spanish
*hola@lluisduran.com*
*www.lluisduran.com*
Barcelona-born Lluís Duran apprenticed under Juli Guasch while studying at the Massana School. He went on to work as a designer for jewelry brands including Montserrat Guardiola, Niessing, Finor, Vasari and Rabat, and now splits his time between his own atelier – opened in 2000 – and freelance collaborations with other Barcelona-based brands. Lluís received the 2008 Catalan Federation of Jewelers, Goldsmiths, and Watchmakers' Innovation and Design Prize. Conceived as portable sculptures, his pieces are chiefly inspired by nature and heavily influenced by early 20th-century design. > p. 26

## LOURDES CARMELO
Spanish
*lourdescarmelo@gmail.com*
*lourdescarmelo.blogspot.com*
A previous runner-up at the Short Message Silver (SMS) Competition at Poland's Legnica Gallery of Art and Barcelona's Enjoia't competition, Lourdes Carmelo harnesses organic and found objects, reworking them to tell new stories. Lourdes learned contemporary jewelry-making at Barcelona's Massana School. She also holds an undergraduate degree in fine art and a postgraduate qualification in museum education from the University of Barcelona. She has exhibited throughout Spain, in Poland and in Mexico, showcasing her work as part of the Joyas Sensacionales project since 2008. > p. 79

## LUIS MÉNDEZ ARTESANOS
Spanish
*info@luismendez.net*
*www.luismendez.net*
Run by a family with over eighty years of experience in the filigree jewelry trade, Luis Méndez Artesanos is an arts and crafts atelier based in Tamames, near Salamanca, Spain. The three owners – brothers Raúl, Luis and Jerónimo – trained under their father, the maestro Luis Méndez Vieira, and strive to combine his classical jewelry-making legacy with a contemporary spin. They have won various distinctions for their work, exhibiting across Spain and at other venues such as the Santa Fe International Folk Art Market in New Mexico. > pp. 32, 33

## MAGALÍ ANIDJAR
Argentinian
*magalianidjar@gmail.com*
*www.magalianidjar.com*
Magali Anidjar's work gives expression to both conscious and unconscious reactions to urban phenomena and day-to-day city life. She is intrigued by the contrast between the architecture of destruction and organic urban development, and often employs wood, found objects and consumer packaging alongside precious and non-precious metals. Magalí trained at Alchimia in Florence, Italy and in Buenos Aires. She has contributed to exhibitions or publications in Buenos Aires, New York, Mexico City and Barcelona. > p. 162

## MANUELA URIBE
Colombian
*manuela.uribe@gmail.com*
Manuela Uribe learned her trade as a jewelry designer at the Academy of Jewelry Art in Rome and the EAFIT University in her hometown of Medellín, where she has also undertaken courses on techniques including gemmology. In 2010 she travelled to Barcelona to complete an enamelling workshop led by Eva Nicolau, Andrea Velázquez Calleja and Karim Oukid. Rich textures and ornate details permeate Manuela's nature-inspired designs, of which she releases two new collections every year. She has also featured in books such as *New Rings.* > p. 152

## MARC MONZÓ
Spanish
*marc@marcmonzo.net*
*www.marcmonzo.net*
The 2006 Catalan Federation of Jewelers, Goldsmiths and Watchmakers Design Prize winner, Barcelona-born Marc Monzó attended the prestigious Massana School. He has had more than twenty-five solo shows worldwide and participated in countless group exhibitions, including at New York's Museum of Decorative Arts and Lisbon's Belém Cultural Centre. He has also taught or lectured at the Massana School, Amsterdam's Gerrit Rietveld Academy and Tokyo's Hiko Mizuno College of Jewelry. His work is displayed in several permanent collections, while publication credits include the monograph *Marc Monzó Jeweler.* > pp. 146, 147

## MAREEN ALBURG DUNCKER
German
*mail@mareenalburg.de*
*www.mareenalburg.com*
After a one-year apprenticeship in Berlin, Mareen Alburg Duncker attended the Burg Giebichenstein University of Art and Design in Halle, Germany, where she now lives and works. Two of her career milestones have come in Halle: First Prize and a showcase at the 2009 Handel Festival and a 2002 solo show. Besides numerous exhibitions throughout Germany, in the Netherlands (at the Marzee Gallery, where her pieces grace the permanent collection) and in Tokyo, Japan, her work features in the books *New Rings* and *500 Earrings.* > pp. 64, 93

## MARÍA CECILIA GÓMEZ BETANCUR
Colombian
*mariatresgatos@gmail.com*
María Cecilia Gómez Betancur turned to jewelry-making following twenty-three years as a French translator and visual artist. The idea of translation continues to underpin her heavily textured, multi-layered work, which she views as a form of Braille that connects tactile and visual experience. Her practice involves reworking cast-off materials into collograph collages, which she then presents in the form of jewelry. A member of the Noi-Joyería collective, María Cecilia trained at EAFIT University, before undertaking miscellaneous courses through the National Apprenticeship Service in her native Medellín. > p. 186

## MARÍA DEL MAR SÁNCHEZ
Spanish
*marsanchezjoyas@gmail.com*
*marsanchezjoyas.wordpress.com*
María del Mar Sánchez enjoys experimenting with and juxtaposing different materials, imbuing her minimalist, deft pieces with a quality redolent of contemporary sculpture. A two-time winner at the Palma de Mallorca Federation of Jewelry Makers and Watchmakers' Joya Mediterránea Competition, María del Mar made her first incursions into jewelry-making in Majorca, at the School of Design and the Spanish Gemmological Institute. She has subsequently studied in Barcelona (including at the Massana School) and in Tarragona, where she now lives. She has twice exhibited at Inhorgenta in Munich. > p. 162

## MARÍA GOTI
Spanish
*info@mariagoti.es*
*www.mariagoti.es*
*mariagoti.blogspot.com*
María Goti learned various jewelry-making techniques at the European Centre of Gemmology and Jewelry Making in her native Oviedo, and also studied resins in Barcelona under Elvira López del Prado. She opened her own atelier in 2006 and sells her pieces online and through collaborations with shops and galleries inside and outside Spain. Combining silver with various effects and textures, María's alluring designs are influenced by her experiences, memories and surroundings, and always bear her trademark: an understated, minimalist finish. > pp. 112, 200

## MARÍA LILIANA RUIZ
Colombian
*contacto@lirujoyas.com*
*www.lirujoyas.com*
*lirujoyas.blogspot.com*
A qualified industrial engineer, Bogotá-born María Liliana Ruiz lived in New York and Germany before moving to Barcelona, Spain, where she began studying art jewelry at the Escola d'Art del Treball in 2008. Major exhibition credits so far include Barcelona's Enjoia't Competition and 'Unexpected Pleasures' at London's Design Museum. María Liliana espouses the notion that jewelry should tell a story, turning the wearer into a stage on which various elements interact. Her pieces figuratively and abstractly interpret stories, memories or emotions. > pp. 95, 160

## MARÍA SOLÓRZANO
Mexican
*maisolorzanojoyeria@gmail.com*
*maijoyeriacontemporanea.blogspot.com*
María Solórzano uses her work to express her perception of the world, the environment, society and human behaviour. She advocates the idea that jewelry need not be precious, making regular use of recycled or recyclable materials. Born in Mexico City, María went to Valencia, Spain, to study industrial design, before moving to Buenos Aires, Argentina, to devote herself to contemporary jewelry. She has exhibited at the International Jewellery Competition in Legnica, Poland, in Argentina and in Mexico (including the solo show 'Iridescencias' at the Pladi Gallery). > p. 168

## MARIANA VISO ROJAS
Venezuelan
*mvisorojas.blogspot.com*
Recipient of the 2007 Prize for Best Technique in the professional division of Barcelona's Enjoia't Contemporary Jewelry Awards, Mariana Viso Rojas trained in Barcelona at the Llotja School and the Catalan Federation of Jewelers, Goldsmiths and Watchmakers. Mariana pinpoints learning about Berber jewelry under Karim Oukid Ouksel as a landmark in her artistic evolution. Although her work has always been instinctive, rather than theoretical, and fuelled by personal emotions, this course marked a spiritual transformation that saw sinuous forms gradually infiltrate her previously rigid, geometric designs. > pp. 30, 63

## MARINA BABIĆ
Bosnian
*marinababic@gmail.com*
*www.marinababic.com*
Educated in Jewelry Arts at George Brown College in Toronto, where she obtained the Gesswein and Shelly Purdy Awards in recognition of her excellence in areas such as technical exploration and design, Marina Babić was awarded a Women's Association of the Mining Industry of Canada Scholarship for Jewellery Design from the Ontario Crafts Council in 2011. Marina transforms natural elements into sculptural jewelry, working mainly in silver and gold, and using a variety of metal-forming methods. Her designs have been exhibited across Canada. > pp. 21, 136

## MARLENE BEYER
German
*marlene@marlene-beyer.de*
*www.marlene-beyer.de*
An exponent of sophisticated feminine design, Marlene Beyer makes jewelry that is playful, fashionable and highly colourful. She adapts everyday objects to create her own pieces, with a particular predilection for plastic, which she self-manufactures and pigments. Marlene attended Düsseldorf's University of Applied Sciences and the Massana School in Barcelona, where she also apprenticed under Marc Monzó. An award-winner at the 20th Legnica International Jewellery Competition, in Poland, she has exhibited in Munich, Amsterdam and Barcelona, and is represented in the 2010 book *Dreaming Jewelry*. > pp. 94, 142

## MARTA CODERQUE
Spanish
*coderque@coderque.com*
*www.coderque.com*
Since starting out in 1998, Marta Coderque has built on her initial studies in jewelry design, stone-setting and CAD 3D modelling with courses in the History of Jewelry through the Spanish National University of Distance Education, Gemmology at the Autonomous University of Madrid and Colored Stone Essentials and Advanced Gemology through the Gemological Institute of America. Predominantly inspired by her surroundings and everyday pleasures, Marta's pieces are impregnated with a spirit of experimentation that drives her ongoing training in different techniques. > pp. 35, 73, 175

## MARTA SÀNCHEZ OMS
Spanish
*hola@masaoms.com*
*www.masaoms.com* | *masaoms.blogspot.com*
Marta Sànchez Oms's upbringing was inextricably linked with handiwork – a budding artisan as a child, her grandfather taught her to fix lights and mend shoes, while she further honed her skills at her father's joinery workshop. The founder of the popular contemporary jewelry forum www.18kt.es, Marta runs her own atelier and showroom in Barcelona, where she studied at the Massana School. Her practice involves fusing personal designs and modern trends with influences including Ancient Egypt, German gemmology, fairy tales and major female figures from history. > pp. 64, 138

## MARTHA VARGAS
Mexican
*marvar98@hotmail.com*
*www.marthavargas.com*
After starting out in the 1980s as a textile designer, Martha Vargas became the highest-paid designer in Mexico, before launching her own jewelry brand in 2000. A multiple award-winner – including twice placing first at the 'Mexico Tercer Milenio' Design Biennial – she has received extensive coverage from magazines including *Vogue*, *Tiempo de Joyas* and *Harper's Bazaar*. Masterfully utilizing wood, bone and lost-wax casting, Martha imbues her pieces with strength and restraint. She regularly draws on elements from the craftmaking tradition of her home state of Michoacán. > p. 27

## MARTIN PAPCÚN
Slovakian
*papcun.net@gmail.com*
*www.papcun.net*
Martin Papcún is intrigued by the twin notions of space and place, delving into them, (re)modelling them – literally and figuratively – and compiling catalogues of related stimuli. After training in metalsmithing in Turnov, the Czech Republic, Martin continued his art education in Prague and Munich. With countless exhibitions under his belt – including several grant-funded site-specific installations in Cleveland, USA, regular appearances at Schmuck and a two-person show at Munich's Akademie Gallery – he graces books such as *New Rings* and collections including Prague's Museum of Decorative Arts. > p. 71

## MARTINA PONT
Spanish
*pontena@hotmail.com*
*curiososecreto.blogspot.com*
Martina Pont has undertaken extensive training in fine art (she holds a BA from the University of Barcelona) and various jewelry techniques – including Japanese lacquer coating, Delft pottery and crystal resin – both in Barcelona and at the Alchimia School in Florence, Italy. Barcelona native Martina has contributed to a long list of group exhibitions at her hometown's Alea Gallery, as well as staging solo shows at the Meko Gallery and Amaranto Joies. Honoured at the 2008 Enjoia't Contemporary Jewelry Awards, she also features in the book *Dreaming Jewelry*. > pp. 52, 200

## MEIRI ISHIDA
Japanese
*fringe2018flower@gmail.com*
*www.meiri-ishida.com*
With a predilection for colour, swirling forms, light materials and a contrast between concentration, continuation and invention, Meiri Ishida describes her work as the poetry of her existence. Meiri followed training at the Tama Art University in her native Tokyo by studying contemporary jewelry at Alchimia, in Florence, Italy. Showcases of her work include the books *500 Necklaces* and *500 Plastic Jewelry Designs* and events such as Schmuck 2006 in Munich, and 'Transfiguration: Japanese Art Jewelry Today' at Tokyo's National Museum of Modern Art. > p. 101

## MIGUEL GASSÓ
German
*mail@rieragasso.com* | *www.rieragasso.com*
After completing metalsmithing and silversmithing apprenticeships, studying industrial design and undergoing an industry placement in his native Germany, Hamelin-born Miguel Gassó obtained a Carl Duisberg Scholarship to attend Barcelona's Massana School. In 1996 Miguel co-founded the Forum Ferlandina Gallery in Barcelona alongside Beatrice Würsch and Montse Rubio, and this was followed in 1999 by the setting-up of the Rieragassó brand, uniting Miguel's expertise in jewelry (including 3D modelling) and industrial design with the experience of his partner Montse Riera, a professional gemmologist. > p. 18

## MIRLA FERNANDES
Brazilian
*mirlaf@gmail.com* | *www.mirlafernandes.com*
*novajoia.blogspot.com*
With a background in biochemistry and fine arts, São Paulo-born Mirla Fernandes studied jewelry design in Pforzheim, Germany. She has enjoyed major showcases in Munich (including Schmuck and a 2005 solo show at the Galerie Biro) and through the exhibition 'Think Twice: New Latin American Jewelry'. A 2010 Prince Claus Award nominee, Mirla employs limited tools for her pieces, focusing instead on her body and movements for inspiration. She regularly utilizes latex, exploring its paint-like qualities when liquid and its wearability and robustness when dry. > p. 78

## MISUN WON
Korean
*misun1110@hotmail.com*
*misunwon.blogspot.com*
In her designs, Misun Won seeks to convey the beauty and symbolic value of *jogakbo*, traditional Korean patchwork. After obtaining a BFA in Precious Metal Design from South Korea's Hangyang University, Misun headed to Scotland to undertake a Masters in Design at Edinburgh College of Art. She has won several awards in Scotland, including a Scottish Arts Council Professional Development Grant and a City of Edinburgh Council Craft Maker Award. Top exhibition credits include SIERAAD in Amsterdam, JOYA in Barcelona and 'Collect' in London. > pp. 152, 214, 218

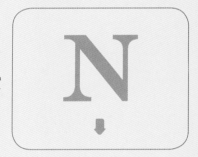

## NADJA SOLOVIEV
German
*nadja.soloviev@gmail.com*
Sandwiched between graduating with honours from the School of Goldsmithing in Pforzheim and embarking on studies at the Academy of Fine Arts in Nuremberg, German designer Nadja Soloviev enjoyed a one-year internship at the Metalab Gallery in Sydney, Australia. She has shown her work in all of these cities, as well as at Melbourne's Pieces of Eight Gallery. Nadja's engaging pieces often combine fine, sterling and oxidized silver. Her recent 'Flat Out' collection deals with the beauty of secrets and keeping them. > p. 117

## NATALIA MILOSZ-PIEKARSKA
Polish
*natalia925@gmail.com* | *ahhness.blogspot.com*
Warsaw native Natalia Milosz-Piekarska trained in gold and silversmithing at Melbourne's RMIT University. Her work has been shown in Australia – including a joint exhibition, 'Bad Beasts Do Not Harm Me', shown in Melbourne and Sydney – and at international venues such as San Francisco's Velvet da Vinci Gallery. Her accolades include a British Council Realise Your Dream Award. Natalia is fascinated by the appeal of charmed objects and the power of belief. Playfully combining unorthodox and traditional approaches, her pieces are endowed with a pervasive sense of spirit and character. > pp. 84, 109

**NICOLAS ESTRADA**
Colombian
*nicolas@amarillojoyas.com*
*www.amarillojoyas.com*
> pp. 35, 102, 131

**NICOLE JACQUARD**
American
*nicolejacquard@gmail.com*
*www.nicolejacquard.com*
Holder of both a BA and an MFA in her native US, Nicole Jacquard was awarded a Fulbright Scholarship which allowed her to travel to Melbourne, Australia, to pursue a second MFA and a PhD in Fine Arts at RMIT University. She has exhibited from Memphis, Tennessee to Riga, Latvia and Herend, Hungary, and contributed to publications such as *500 Silver Jewelry Designs* and *The Best of the 500 Series*. Replete with subtle details and fusing orthodox and non-traditional methods, Nicole's pieces aim to render ordinary events extraordinary. > pp. 193, 205

**NOEL GUYOMARC'H**
Canadian
*www.galerienoelguyomarch.com*
Noel Guyomarc'h has been working in the field of jewelry-making for over twenty years. In 1996 he opened his own gallery in Montreal, Canada, where he has commissioned, promoted and organized more than seventy solo and group exhibitions. Regularly invited to serve on exhibition juries and to speak at conferences, he has also been an advisor to the Montreal Museum of Fine Arts for several years. In 2002 he joined the board of the Montreal Jewelry School, serving as its president from 2006–2011. A member of numerous national and international associations, he has featured in an extensive range of publications. > pp. 8–9

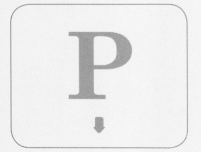

**PACO RIVAS**
Spanish
*pcko.rivas@gmail.com*
*pacorivas.blogspot.com*
A fine art graduate from the University of Barcelona, Granada-born Paco Rivas worked as a graphic and costume designer before travelling to New York, where he began building PMMA models for an architecture firm. After designing pendants for a rock band in 2007, Paco turned his focus to jewelry-making, applying classical carving techniques to his explorations of mythology, animals and nature. As well as events such as JOYA in Barcelona and Madrid's Iberjoya, he has featured in Spain's *Contemporary Jewellery Yearbook 2011*. > p. 172

**PATRICIA LEMAIRE**
French
*contact@spo-creations.com*
*www.spo-creations.com | blog.spo-creations.com*
The relationship between object and body and the body's transformation in space are the constants that guide the work of French artist Patricia Lemaire. Whether a form of expression or a means of telling a story, her distinctive, diverse pieces always bear the hallmark of true jewelry. Now a resident of Clamart, just outside Paris, Patricia trained in applied arts in Metz and decorative arts in Strasbourg. Her work is found in numerous galleries, design stores and collections, and she frequently collaborates with fashion and haute couture designers. > pp. 21, 177

**PAULA ESTRADA**
Colombian
*paula.estrada@almapropia.com*
*www.almapropia.com*
An award-winning industrial designer honoured with Colombia's prestigious Steel Pencil Award, Paula Estrada is drawn to jewelry-making's communicative potential. She sees it as a perfect three-dimensional field, allowing her to channel multiple influences – including architecture, nature, contemporary art and her travels – into her concepts, processes and disciplines. Featured in several major Colombian design magazines and the book *New Rings*, Paula studied industrial design at the Pontifical Bolivarian University in Medellín. She embarked on metalwork studies at Barcelona's El Taller in 2010. > p. 31

**PETER HOOGEBOOM**
Dutch
*hoogeboom@upcmail.nl*
*www.peterhoogeboom.nl*
Educated at Amsterdam's Gerrit Rietveld Academy, Peter Hoogeboom combines ceramics and contemporary jewelry in his original concept creations, often displaying new kinds of wearability. Peter has won and been nominated for multiple awards, notably Italy's Cominelli Foundation Award for Contemporary Jewellery, the European Prize for Applied Arts and Australia's Gold Coast International Ceramic Art Award. Showcased in the books *Dreaming Jewelry* and *Art Jewelry Today 3*, his work has been exhibited in the solo show 'Sieraarden' in Amsterdam and 'A Bit of Clay on the Skin' at MAD, New York. > p. 140

**PETRA CLASS**
German
*petra.class@gmail.com*
*www.petraclass.com*
San Francisco resident Petra Class studied art history and philosophy at the University of Stuttgart (her hometown) and attended the State College for Glass and Jewelry in Neugablonz, Germany. Books such as *New Rings* and *500 Earrings* have published her pieces. Comparing her practice to a jazz melody or an abstract landscape, Petra delights in reformulating a reduced range of elements to forge innovative – yet always wearable – solutions, often featuring unusual textural contrasts. She is fascinated by the painterly colours prevalent in natural gemstones. > pp. 29, 41

**PILAR COTTER**
Spanish
*pilar-cotter.blogspot.com*
Counting Manon van Kouswijk amongst her major influences, Pilar Cotter draws her creative thrust from everyday objects and in particular from conversations. Her recent pieces explore illusions and mirages, truth and lies, and the complexity of synthesis. After studying fine art in Tenerife, Pilar pursued jewelry design at the Massana School in Barcelona, where she has also won prizes at Enjoia't and enjoyed a debut solo show at the Amaranto Gallery. Other showcases have come in Munich and Detroit, as well as in Carles Codina's book *The New Jewelry*. > p. 137

**PILAR GARRIGOSA**
Spanish
*pilar@garrigosa.com*
*www.garrigosa.com*
Pilar Garrigosa followed studies under Carles Codina at the Massana School with a course at the Llotja School, also in Barcelona. Her breakthrough year came in 2000, being shortlisted at Inhorgenta in Munich and winning the Paola and Lucia Molin Award in Padua, where she has repeatedly exhibited over the years. Rationalism and sensuality coalesce in Pilar's work, which juxtaposes exuberant jewels full of personality with geometric metal forms. Her pieces appear in *New Rings* and the *Contemporary Jewellery Yearbook 2011*. > pp. 15, 58

**PILI ÁNGEL LOSADA**
Colombian
*pili_angel@hotmail.com*
*www.piliangel.com*
With a background in marketing, Pili Ángel Losada is attracted to jewelry's potential as a vehicle for personal expression. Her jewelry reflects her passion for freedom and arousing the senses. Primarily employing silver, bronze, copper, raw stones, beads and silk ribbons, her colourful pieces pay tribute to traditional artisanship, interweaving stories and highlighting the value of the handmade. A resident of the Colombian capital of Bogotá, Pili holds an MA in Fashion Management and took part in the first Braincelona event in Barcelona. > p. 190

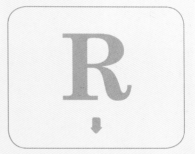

**RIKE BARTELS**
German
*rike@rikebartels.com*
*www.rikebartels.com*
Born in Munich, Rike Bartels trained first in Spain, then in the Black Forest, Germany, and finally in Italy, in particular crediting Manfred Bischoff for much of what she knows about art, jewelry and many other things besides. Featured in a two-person exhibition at Munich's Isabella Hund Gallery, Rike has displayed her creations throughout Europe, including at London's Victoria & Albert Museum and Prague's Museum of Applied Arts. Publications include *New Rings*, *Art Meets Jewellery: 20 Years of Galerie Slavik Vienna* and *Masters: Gold*. > pp. 15, 56, 61, 62

**ROC MAJORAL & ABRIL RIBERA**
Spanish
*info@majoral.com*
*www.majoral.com*
Roc Majoral and Abril Ribera are both products of the studio of Enric Majoral, where they continue to practice. In their independent work, they are driven by a passion for discovery and experimentation, regularly utilizing cutting-edge technologies and materials. The compass guiding their jewelry, however, always remains the same: to highlight the beauty of the wearer. Their work has been showcased in numerous publications – including *New Rings* and the magazines *Vogue*, *Elle* and *Arte y Joya* – and at top exhibitions in Barcelona and Formentera, Spain. > pp. 28, 43, 201, 212

### RODRIGO ACOSTA ARIAS
Argentinian
*rodrigoacostacrea@gmail.com*
*www.rodrigoacostarias.blogspot.com*
Rodrigo Acosta Arias holds degrees in product and fashion design from the National University of Cuyo in Mendoza and the National University of Buenos Aires respectively. After working for prestigious Argentinian jewelry brand Sibilia, he moved to Valencia, Spain, to hone his technique with a course in art jewelry at the Higher School of Art and Design. Rodrigo enjoys hybridizing objects to find common ground or forge something new. He often draws on his experience in fashion to find forms that fit the body. > p. 70

### RUDEE TANCHAROEN
Thai
*contact@rudeetancharoen.com*
*www.rudeetancharoen.com*
Bangkok-born Rudee Tancharoen expresses the purity and fragility of life through pieces that often combine a naive aesthetic with hints of irony. Rudee embarked on her jewelry-making studies at the Alchimia School in Florence, Italy, completing an exchange programme at the University of Applied Arts in Idar-Oberstein, Germany, in 2007, her graduation year. The recipient of the Second Prize and the Organizers' Special Award at the 2007 Silver Festival in Legnica, Poland, she appears in publications including *The Compendium Finale of Contemporary Jewellers*. > p. 113

### RYAN DE JAGER
South African
*miyagi.dejager@gmail.com*
*outdiebox.blogspot.com*
Chiefly driven by the pursuit of play, Ryan de Jager frequently combines silver and other traditional metalwork materials with old toys, thereby fostering nostalgia and allowing people to connect with his pieces on several levels. He also enjoys embedding identity into materials that might otherwise be deemed worthless. After a first incursion into the field at Cape Town's Ruth Prowse School of Art, Ryan went on to undertake a degree in Jewellery Design and Manufacture at the Cape Peninsula University of Technology. > p. 207

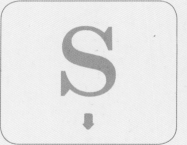

### SALVADOR MALLOL
Spanish
*verdi@mallol.com*
*www.mallol.com*
With over twenty years' experience, Salvador Mallol trained in gemmology and jewelry-making in Barcelona, where he now runs one of his two shops (the other is in nearby Sant Cugat). He was recognized for his efforts at Barcelona's Enjoia't Competition in 2006. Often combining precious metals with recycled and industrial materials, Salvador derives huge pleasure from demonstrating how much can be done with limited means. Displaying his own brand of ingenuity, he attributes the inspiration behind his work to chance. > pp. 19, 63, 211

### SAMUEL SAAVEDRA
Spanish
*operajoies@telefonica.net*
A winner at the 1994–95 Enjoia't competition, Samuel Saavedra majored in metalsmithing at Barcelona's Llotja School. In 2010 he was awarded the title of Master Artisan by the Government of Catalonia. Samuel's geometric designs eschew overblown ornamentation in favour of a lighter, more essential form of beauty. They have made their way into publications such as *New Rings* and exhibitions including ¡Ojo! An Exhibition of Spanish Contemporary Jewellery' in Manchester, England and the solo show 'Geometria en Joc' at Barcelona's Alea Gallery. > p. 139

### SANDRA PONTNOU FERRER
Spanish
*sandrapofe@yahoo.es*
*joiaespai.blogspot.com*
With a background in geology, which she studied at the Autonomous University of Barcelona, Sandra Pontnou Ferrer was drawn to jewelry by her passion for gems. Indeed, she personally sources precious and semi-precious stones for use in the vast majority of her pieces, which are characterized by pure lines and geometric forms. Sandra learned her trade through a veritable multitude of courses in Barcelona, including at the Llotja School, the Espiral School and the Catalan Federation of Jewelers, Goldsmiths and Watchmakers. > p. 152

### SARAH WEST
American
*sarahwestdesigns@gmail.com*
*sarahwestdesigns.com*
Fascinated by electrical towers, line drawings and maps, Sarah West mobilizes memories to establish links between the past and present. Vinyl from old LPs joins more traditional materials such as silver and steel in her pieces. Seattle-born, Sarah went to the North Bennet Street School in Boston, before obtaining a BFA from East Carolina University in Greenville, North Carolina, graduating magna cum laude. She has picked up manifold distinctions, including a prize-winning appearance at the 2010 National Student Juried Exhibition and a 2011 NICHE Student Award. > p. 98

### SAYUMI YOKOUCHI
Japanese
*sayumi6@gmail.com*
*www.sayumiyokouchi.com*
Tokyo-born Sayumi Yokouchi made her first silver ring while at high school in her home country. She delights in the transformative possibilities afforded by different materials and objects. After moving to the US in 1990, Sayumi studied metal design at California College of the Arts and SUNY New Paltz, before opening her own studio in Brooklyn, New York. Her pieces are displayed in the books *New Rings*, *Jewellery from Natural Materials* and Lark Books' *500 Earrings*. > p. 153

### SELMA LEAL
Brazilian
*learagroup@gmail.com*
*selmaleal.blogspot.com*
São Paulo native Selma Leal has amassed the bulk of her training, major exhibitions and career milestones in Barcelona, Spain, including numerous courses at the Escola d'Art del Treball and the Llotja School. In 2009 she opened the Atelier Leara in the city. The winner of the First Bagués-Masriera International Enamel Award, Selma has been shortlisted for the Tahitian Pearl Trophy and Swarovski's Create Your Style Awards. Her designs reflect the joy of freedom and the simplicity of life and nature. > p. 166

### SENAY AKIN
Turkish
*info@senayakin.com*
*www.senayakin.com*
Senay Akin views her pieces as three-dimensional narratives weaving a story inspired by literature, the materials they are made of and the cultures she has experienced through her travels. After pursuing photography at the Mimar Sinan University of Fine Arts in Istanbul – where she had her first solo exhibition – Senay learned jewelry design at the School of Arts and Crafts in Vicenza, Italy. She has featured in the JOYA Barcelona Contemporary Jewelry Week, the book *New Rings* and the magazines *Elle*, *Trendsetter* and *Maison Française*. > pp. 106, 174, 177

### SHARON SCHAFFNER
American
*shaz27@chisp.net*
Nature, current issues and travel inspire the engaging work of Houston-born artist Sharon Schaffner. Sharon earned a BFA in her hometown and has been designing jewelry for almost forty years. Now based in Denver, Colorado, she has taken part in exhibitions in places including Takayama, Japan; the National Archaeological Museum of Tarragona, Spain (the four-person show 'From Memory to Creation. Order and Chaos'); and Barcelona. Publication credits include *Contemporary Enameling: Art and Technique* and the Spanish magazines *Arte y Joya* and *Eurodesign*. > pp. 112, 172

### SHU-LIN WU
Taiwanese
*shulin_wu@hotmail.com | www.shulinwu.com*
Taiwanese designer Shu-Lin Wu graduated from the School of Decorative Arts in Strasbourg, France. A 2008 winner of Comité Colbert's Young Designers Competition, she exhibited solo in Lappeenranta, Finland in 2006. In 2011 she received a travel grant from Taiwan's National Culture and Arts Foundation and attended two major ceramic jewelry-related exhibitions in the US: at Pewabic Pottery, Detroit and MAD, New York, respectively. Her increasing shift towards incorporating clay – symbolizing her native soil and culture – embodies the coming together of Western and Eastern influences in her work. > p. 118

### SIM LUTTIN
Australian
*simluttin@gmail.com | www.simluttin.com*
After a BFA at the RMIT University, Melbourne native Sim Luttin completed an MA in Metalsmithing and Jewelry Design at Indiana University. Major achievements include being commissioned to create the Emeritus Medal by the Australia Council for the Arts, solo exhibitions in Melbourne and Sydney and numerous prestigious group shows. Her pieces – which probe into the symbiotic relationship between objects and memory – feature in the collections of the Marzee Gallery in the Netherlands and the Art Gallery of South Australia, as well as several Lark Books volumes. > p. 192

### SÒNIA SERRANO
Spanish
*sonia.serrano.p@gmail.com*
*soniaserranop.blogspot.com*
Sònia Serrano shares her time between designing, exhibiting across her hometown of Barcelona – including at the Alea Gallery and the home of FAD (Fostering Arts and Design) – and teaching at the Escola d'Art del Treball. She majored in sculpture at the University of Barcelona and trained as a jeweler at the Llotja School. The cornerstone of Sònia's work is a passion for experimentation and strikingly unusual combinations. Conceived as miniature wearable sculptures, her pieces are at once highly playful and easy to play with. > p. 209

## SOPHIA GEORGIOPOULOU
Greek
*kosmimata@gmail.com*
*www.kosmimata.com*
A classics graduate who holds a PhD in Byzantine Literature from Harvard University, Sophia Georgiopoulou taught in that field until 2004, before qualifying as a goldsmith and opening an atelier, Kosmimata, in her native Athens in 2010. Sophia draws heavily on Hellenistic, Roman and Byzantine influences in her work, utilizing the ancient technique of granulation to craft objects of timeless beauty. She works mainly in gold and silver, although three of her metal clay designs were selected for the *PMC Guild Annual 5.* > pp. 38, 50

......................

## SOPHIE BOUDUBAN
Swiss
*sbouduban@sunrise.ch*
Employing metals, glass and even bone, Sophie Bouduban's pieces dwell poetically on issues relating to death and mortality. The recipient of a Swiss Federal Grant of Applied Arts in 1994, Sophie attended Geneva's School of Applied Arts. Featured in the *Dictionnaire International du Bijou*, she has exhibited throughout her homeland – including at Lausanne's Museum of Design and Contemporary Applied Arts (MUDAC) and Geneva's Museum of Art and History – and in the US (including SOFA), where she is represented by New York's Charon Kransen Arts. > p. 73

......................

## SU KROKER
German
*su-design@hetnet.nl*
*www.schmuckvirus.com*
In 2008, the sight of burrs sticking to children's clothes in a park inspired Su Kroker to launch the 'Schmuckvirus' concept, in which she spreads happiness by passing on 'jewelry viruses' at trade fairs worldwide. Her one-of-a-kind pieces are highly structural, flowing and delicately crocheted, offering an escape into a fairy-tale world. Born in Stuttgart, Su apprenticed as a silversmith before learning metal design in Hildesheim, Germany. In 1997 she undertook a Leonardo da Vinci work placement in Delft, the Netherlands, later establishing her atelier in the Dutch town of Blokzijl. > pp. 143, 174

......................

## SUSAN MAY
British
*susan@susanmay.org* | *www.susanmay.org*
Susan May savours the processes through which her pieces take shape, regardless of how far they depart from her preliminary ideas, which she tends to sketch out in busy urban settings. An experimental, intuitive designer boasting over twenty-five years of experience, Susan graces several top jewelry books and regularly exhibits at London's renowned 'Collect' show. Exhibition highlights include 'Creation 11' at London's Goldsmiths' Hall, for which a DVD documentary showcasing the twelve participants was produced, and shows at Velvet da Vinci, San Francisco, and MAD, New York. > pp. 114, 136

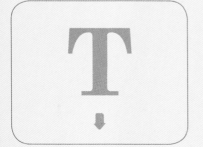

## TANIA SKLYAR
Ukrainian
*contact@tania-sklyar.de* | *www.tania-sklyar.de*
Recycling and breathing new life into used objects are key motifs of the work of Berlin-based Tania Sklyar, who trained in her hometown of Odessa, the Ukraine. This approach is consistent with her interest in deviating from the beaten track and reclaiming childhood secrets and memories. She recognizes the unusual influence on her work of photographer Joel-Peter Witkin's explorations of physical deformation and death. She has contributed to several magazines, the book *New Rings*, the JOYA Barcelona Contemporary Jewelry Week and Berlin's RestCycling Art Festival. > p. 81

......................

## TERRY WARE
American
*www.terryware.net*
Terry Ware is entranced by the magic produced by the reincarnation of earthly materials. She compares her practice to the way in which a nest is gradually formed from twigs or leaves are reborn by bonding with the soil. An awareness of the relationship between culture, history and art underlies her work. An art historian by training, Terry is self-taught as a jeweler and has been running her own studio since 1998. She was born in Los Angeles and presently operates out of New York. > p. 141

......................

## THERESA BURGER
South African
*tweebi@gmail.com*
*www.theresaburger.com*
After finishing undergraduate studies in her native Cape Town, Theresa Burger moved to Dublin, Ireland to undertake an MA at the National College of Art and Design. A 2011 Crafts Council of Ireland Future Maker Award winner, she has appeared at numerous top Irish exhibitions, including 'Design Tree' in late 2010. Theresa's work stretches the established boundaries of jewelry-making, combining digital design and rapid prototyping with artisanal traditions. She draws heavily on contemporary architecture and the shapes and colours of the Zulu Nation. > pp. 100, 186

......................

## TIFFANY ROWE
British-Swiss
*tiffany.rowe@crea-tiff.ch*
*www.crea-tiff.ch* | *creatiffbijoux.tumblr.com*
The offbeat British-Swiss designer Tiffany Rowe studied biology at university. A Geneva native and resident, she is fascinated by molecules and spheres, which she often reproduces through organic round shapes in her work. Designed to be worn 'backwards', the pieces in Tiffany's 'Recto Verso' earring series draw their inspiration from the elliptical trajectories of electrons. A great admirer of contemporary art and photography, she regularly contributes to all kinds of artistic projects. > p. 224

......................

## TINA LILIENTHAL
German
*info@tinalilienthal.com*
*www.tinalilienthal.com*
A graduate of London's Royal College of Art, Tina Lilienthal's fabulously edgy designs have earned her wide acclaim and distinctions including the Marzee Prize and the Goldsmiths' Company's First Prize for Fashion Jewellery. Displaying an unorthodox mixture of materials and iconography, Tina's pieces drive to the core of popular culture and human nature, while exploring issues such as love, desire and loss. They have made their way into exhibitions across the UK, including notably 'The Watkins Era' at CAA (Contemporary Applied Arts) in London. > p. 130

## TORE SVENSSON
Swedish
*tore.s@comhem.se*
*www.toresvensson.com*
Tore Svensson's geometric creations are predominantly worked in steel, a material that particularly lends itself to his exploration of different surfaces – through methods such as hammering, gilding and etching – and the interplay of weight and lightness. Tore attended Västerberg Art School and the University of Gothenburg, both in his native Sweden. More than thirty-five years of experience have taken him to myriad top galleries worldwide, and he is showcased in various books, including the monograph *Tore Svensson*. He was awarded the 1999 Bavarian State Prize. > p. 62

......................

## TOVE KNUTS
Swedish
*info@toveknuts.se*
*www.toveknuts.se*
After a first taste of silversmithing in 1991, Swedish designer Tove Knuts later enrolled in a metal arts programme at Konstfack, the University College of Arts, Crafts and Design in Stockholm. Having honed her skills in Prague and Auckland, she has exhibited from Tallinn in Estonia to Legnica in Poland and Amsterdam in the Netherlands. Tove is fascinated by the origin of pearls as a self-defence mechanism for oysters. She attempts to capture this organic sense of growth in her pearl earrings, which resemble chains of molecules. > p. 93

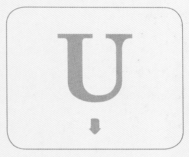

## ULLA & MARTIN KAUFMANN
German
*ulla-martin-kaufmann@t-online.de*
*www.ulla-martin-kaufmann.de*
Hailing from Hildesheim, Germany, Ulla and Martin Kaufmann carried out gold and silversmithing apprenticeships before spending periods in Norway and France. Otherwise self-taught, they have been designing jewelry freelance for over forty years. The subjects of a monograph – *Ulla + Martin Kaufmann: Different From* – produced to accompany the exhibition of the same name held in Nuremberg, Germany, the pair have won the Bavaria and Hesse State Prizes and the iF Product Design Award. Forged bands form the basis for their elegant gold and silver creations. > p. 208

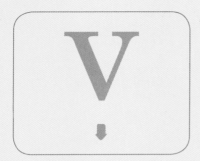

## VALDIS BROZE
Latvian
*gallery@putti.lv*
*www.putti.lv*
Valdis Broze was born and educated in the Latvian capital of Riga, studying metal design at the School of Applied Arts and then gaining a BA and MA at the Art Academy of Latvia. He has enjoyed a solo exhibition ('Ekstra') at Riga's Putti Gallery and contributed to a show on Baltic conceptual jewelry at the National Museum of Decorative Arts in Madrid. Striking colours and enamel craftwork are the signature trademarks of Valdis's sculptural creations. A lifelong love of big cities also informs his craft. > pp. 85, 107

. . . . . . . . . . . . . . . . . . . . . .

## VANESSA LEU
Taiwanese
*info@vanessaleu.com | www.vanessaleu.com*
Los Angeles-based Vanessa Leu's spirituality-infused work engages with social causes and the relationship between inner and outer beauty. Conceived as talismans, her pieces utilize eco-friendly materials, reclaimed metals and conflict-free diamonds. Named a 2010 JCK Rising Star, Vanessa studied gemmology in her native Taiwan, before attending the Gemological Institute of America. Honoured with numerous Chinese government distinctions, she has been featured on Taiwanese radio and Chinese and US television, including the hit shows *Grey's Anatomy*, *American Idol* and *Heroes*. > pp. 39, 79

. . . . . . . . . . . . . . . . . . . . . .

## VÍCTOR SALDARRIAGA
Colombian
*www.lasierpe.net*
Víctor Saldarriaga trained at the Bolivarian Pontifical University in his native Medellín, working at various independent ateliers before opening up his own business in the city. He is certified by the Colombian Institute for Technical Standards and Certification (ICONTEC). Víctor is unable to pin down a specific source of inspiration for his work beyond his general surroundings. Organic and structural effects make their way into his pieces, which tend to use classical materials and aim, above all, to spark a reaction in the beholder. > pp. 109, 194

. . . . . . . . . . . . . . . . . . . . . .

## VIKKI KASSIORAS
Australian
*vikki@vikkikassioras.com.au*
*www.vikkikassioras.com.au*
*vikkikassioras.blogspot.com*
Vikki Kassioras fashions myth-inspired narratives upon which viewers can map their own experiences. She attempts to connect past and present through reference to a collective body of knowledge while fostering personal bonds between work, wearer and viewer. Vikki trained in fine art gold and silversmithing at the RMIT University in her native Melbourne. Exhibition highlights include shows at e.g.etal and Craft Victoria in her hometown, and Talente 2001 in Munich. > pp. 57, 175, 185, 212

## VINA RUST
American
*verust@hotmail.com*
*www.vinarust.com*
A BFA holder from the University of Washington, where she garnered the Marilyn Werby Rabinovitch Memorial Award, Vina Rust has exhibited extensively, including in her current home of Seattle and at 'The Pendant Show' at San Francisco's Velvet da Vinci. *The Best of the 500 Series*, *New Rings* and *Metalsmith* magazine are just some of her publication credits. Vina's recent work gives voice to the wonder of botanical illustrations and photomicrographs, with an emphasis on the musicality of cellular structures. > pp. 104, 105

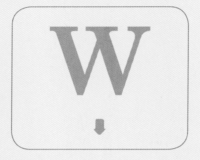

## WALKA STUDIO
(Claudia Betancourt & Nano Pulgar)
Chilean
*www.walka.cl*
UNESCO Chile has recognized the environmentally-aware efforts of Claudia Betancourt and Nano Pulgar, the pair behind Walka Studio, and their contribution to traditional Chilean handicrafts. They have earned grants from the Chilean National Culture Council and showcased their pieces in Mexico, Australia, Chile, the UK, India (at the World Crafts Council) and New York's Museum of Arts and Design (MAD). Issues such as identity, religion, the commoditization of crafts and the overlap between art, crafts and design inform their work. > pp. 42, 96, 143, 164, 174

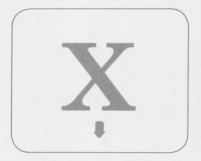

## XANATH LAMMOGLIA BUSTAMANTE
Mexican
*contacto@xanathlammoglia.com*
*www.xanathlammoglia.com*
Following five years as a professional ballet dancer, Mexico City-born Xanath Lammoglia Bustamante studied design in Mexico and at Milan's Marangoni Institute, where she undertook a one-year fashion course. In 2000 she co-founded Bala Studio with Andrés Amaya. Besides gracing various international exhibitions, Xanath has appeared in books including *Diseño: México*, *Sex Design*, *Young Designers Americas* and publications in Russia, Italy, Mexico, the UK – whose *Wallpaper* magazine named her Young Designer of the Year in 2004 – and the US. > p. 25

## XAVIER MONCLÚS
Spanish
*xinesmonclus@yahoo.es*
Educated at Barcelona's Massana School, Xavier Monclús uses jewelry to mould a personal world and express his own viewpoint, utilizing a highly lucid narrative language and a variety of tones. His collage-like painted pieces commonly combine silver, bronze, wood and found objects. Xavier had a solo exhibition, 'De Pinguins van Amsterdam', at Amsterdam's Rob Koudijs Gallery in 2011. He has also participated in major shows in Italy – including at the Le Arti Orafe Gallery in Lucca and the Oratory of San Rocco in Padua. > p. 129

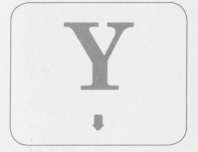

## YAEL SERFATY & TAL SALOMON
Israeli
*yaeltal.j.design@gmail.com*
Yael & Tal is a jewelry studio established in 2011 by Yael Serfaty and Tal Salomon, two graduates of the Jewelry Design Department at Israel's Shenkar College of Engineering and Design, in Ramat Gan. Yael also boasts an MA in Luxury Design from the prestigious Creative Academy in Milan, Italy. The duo's original collections, which channel small details to exploit jewelry's potential to immortalize moments and memories, have appeared in several Israeli exhibitions (including at the Geological Museum in Ramat HaSharon), magazines and fashion websites. > p. 210

. . . . . . . . . . . . . . . . . . . . . .

## YOKO SHIMIZU
Japanese
*yokoshimizu8@gmail.com*
*yokoshimizu.alchimia.it*
A law graduate from Keio University in Tokyo, Yoko Shimizu attended the Alchimia School in Florence, Italy, where she has taught since 2006. Showcases across Europe and in the US, Israel, Japan and Korea and appearances in books including five different Lark Books titles attest to her renown. She also won the 2006 Best Stand Award at 'Origin: The London Craft Fair'. Yoko is fascinated by the varying types of transformation involved in the production of jewelry, whose components lose and gain something at the same time. > p. 110

. . . . . . . . . . . . . . . . . . . . . .

I always dreamed of writing a book, of expressing my feelings, thoughts and my personal way of life through this medium. Although not a piece of writing as such, this is my second volume dedicated to the passion that has become my guiding force: jewelry, an art that has informed and enriched my thoughts and provided me with a beautiful and noble vehicle with which to engage with the world.

Exactly twelve years ago, I picked up my first jewelry-making tool at Barcelona's Llotja School. Thanks to the passion for this wonderful discipline conveyed by my teachers, both there and later at the Massana School, what I had expected to be nothing more than a hobby soon became my profession and a passion of my own.

What I most enjoyed about putting together this book was the opportunity to discover and shine a spotlight on the work of other jewelers all around the world, many of whom I now count among my friends. They are fellow metal artisans who, like me, have chosen to adopt this challenging but highly rewarding art as a way of life.

For me, this book represents a way of paying tribute to a demanding, solitary craft that requires many hours of reflection and learning, of developing and experimenting with ideas. Although there can be setbacks along the way, this practice is a source of endless satisfaction, none greater than when you see a customer proudly sporting one of your designs.

I would like to express my sincerest thanks to everybody who made this book, of which I feel so proud, possible. First of all, my parents, Mauricio and Lina, who have given me unconditional support, a vital aid in navigating the tricky waters of artistic creation. Catalina, my dear sister, has shown me that no goal is too big, taught me that you can achieve anything you can imagine, and set an example with her effort and dedication; her influence in my life cannot be overstated. I am particularly indebted to Andrea Velázquez, Karim Oukid and Paula Estrada, my workshop colleagues, for sharing their expertise and friendship with me on a daily basis; to Carles Codina, my erstwhile teacher and now a good friend, for always believing in me; to Pilar Garrigosa, my guardian angel and an exceptional jeweler, for opening some doors that I might otherwise have struggled to get through; to Juan Cardosa, for bringing everything together and sprinkling his magic on this book; to Joaquín Canet, my publisher, for believing in a foreign jeweler and putting his faith in me for this ambitious project; to Inma Alavedra, for everything she has done to make this volume perfect; to Carolina Hornauer and Noel Guyomarc'h for their contributions, which do a wonderful job of framing these pages; and to the magical city of Barcelona, where I pitched up some twelve years ago and which has since become my home, for always allowing me to be just the person I wanted to be.

And finally, thanks to all the jewelers who have believed in me and this project for granting me access to their creations, many of which are displayed in these pages.

# ACKNOWLEDGMENTS

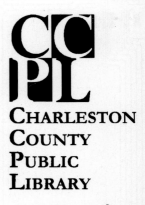